Zion-Benton
Public Library District
Zion, Illinois 60099

DEMCO

The
5
Reasons
Why We Overeat

The 5 *Reasons Why We Overeat*

How to Develop a Long-Term Weight-Control Plan That's Right for You

Cynthia G. Last, Ph.D.

A Birch Lane Press Book
Published by Carol Publishing Group

A Birch Lane Press Book
Published by Carol Publishing Group
Birch Lane Press is a registered trademark of Carol Communications, Inc.

Editorial, sales and distribution, rights and permissions inquiries should be
addressed to Carol Publishing Group, 120 Enterprise Avenue, Secaucus, N.J.
07094.

In Canada: Canadian Manda Group, One Atlantic Avenue, Suite 105, Toronto,
Ontario, M6K 3E7

Carol Publishing Group books may be purchased in bulk at special discounts for
sales promotion, fund-raising, or educational purposes. Special editions can be
created to specifications. For details, contact Special Sales Department, Carol
Publishing Group, 120 Enterprise Avenue, Secaucus, N.J. 07094.

Manufactured in the United States of America
10 9 8 7 6 5 4 3 2 1

Library of Congress Cataloging-in-Publication Data

Last, Cynthia G.
    The five reasons why we overeat : how to develop a long-term
  weight-control plan that's right for you / Cynthia G. Last.
        p.   cm.
  "A Birch Lane Press book."
  Includes index.
  ISBN 1–55972–479–X
  1. Weight loss—Psychological aspects.   2. Compulsive eating.
  I. Title.
  RM222.2.L35   1998
  616.85'26—dc21   98–34216
                                                        CIP

Contents

Disclaimer

This book explores medical issues and dietary guidelines. Neither the author of this book nor its publishers assume any responsibility. Before beginning any dietary, weight-loss, or exercise program, always consult your physician.

The
5
Reasons
Why We Overeat

Introduction:
Why One Diet Doesn't Fit All

At forty-nine, Gail has been overweight for more than thirty years. She's seen a lot of different diets come and go, and has tried most of them: low fat, high protein, low carbohydrate, the "grapefruit diet," the "cabbage diet," the "water diet," diets named after doctors, diets named after cities.

Regardless of which method she uses, Gail always gains the weight back. As a result, she has three different wardrobes—her skinny clothes (size 12) for when she's at the low end of the scale, her chubby clothes (size 14) for when she's gained some of the weight back, and her fat clothes (size 16) for when she's gained all of the weight back.

Now Gail's having trouble fitting into her fat clothes, but refuses to go shopping. She can't face the fact that despite all of her efforts, she weighs *even more* than before.

Gail's story is not unique. Millions of men and women have similar weight-loss histories, punctuated by highs and lows, peaks and valleys. For these people—and probably for you too—permanent weight control, where one's ideal weight is obtained and maintained, seems elusive.

Perhaps the hardest part of my work with overweight people is convincing them that focusing on *what* they eat is not the solution to their weight problem.

The diet industry has a long history of promoting diet and nutritional changes as the key to weight loss. Being influenced by this idea, most of us have gone from one diet to the next, following the fads religiously, hoping for a miracle—that one special diet that allows us to lose the weight and keep it off forever.

If a low-fat diet doesn't do it, maybe a low-carbohydrate one will. If low carbohydrates don't work, switch to a high-protein diet. While some of these diets have helped us to drop a few pounds or even more, none of them have enabled us to keep the weight off permanently.

There is no question that a reduced-calorie diet of almost any type can help us become thin. Moreover, in today's "eating environment" it should be especially easy to follow a low-calorie weight-loss program. Reduced-calorie foods are readily available in our supermarkets, everything from prepared frozen entrées to low-fat brownies that can satisfy the cravings of even the most ardent chocoholic. Most restaurants offer low-calorie meal choices, and even those who travel frequently can arrange for in-flight meals that are reduced in calories.

Yet despite these modern conveniences, as a nation we are fatter, not thinner, than ever before. In fact, with the exception of a few island populations in the Pacific, the United States contains the heaviest people on Earth. In fact, some experts argue that we may be the fattest society that has ever existed in the history of the world.

Research studies show that only a small percentage of overweight adults who try to lose weight through reduced-calorie diets ever reach their ideal weight. Besides disappointing results from short-term weight loss, the news for long-term maintenance of weight loss is even more discouraging: Of the few who do achieve their goal, almost all will regain the weight lost over time. In other words, in the battle against obesity, *relapse is the rule,* not the exception.

Apparently, we aren't able to stick with reduced-calorie eating for the long run. We return to our old eating habits, sometimes quickly, sometimes slowly, but in either event, inevitably. Why can't we simply eat less?

Although almost any type of controlled-calorie approach to eating will be successful for weight control, you must follow the plan for it to be effective. That statement may sound obvious and a bit simplistic; unfortunately, the reasons people have trouble limiting their food intake for the long run are actually rather complex. There are factors, other than *what* we eat, that are sabotaging our efforts to lose weight. The factors are psychological and are different for different people.

As long as our focus remains on what we eat, rather than why we eat, we will continue to be an overweight nation. To get control of our eating and our weight, we must come to terms with the real underlying reasons why we overeat.

In doing so, no single diet method will be effective for all of us. The treatment of overeating must be tailored specifically to the individual, with different methods used for different people. Moreover, the treatments must be psychological in nature, designed to directly address the specific psychological factors that cause overeating.

The idea of individualized psychological treatments for weight loss differs dramatically from the "one diet fits all" mentality that has dominated the diet and weight-loss field for nearly a century. However, it is this mentality that is responsible for your inability to achieve long-term weight control. Permanent weight control cannot be obtained with diets, and there is no one single approach to weight loss that will work for everybody.

Despite the fact that "miracle diets" are often illogical or downright dangerous, such programs generally have sold quite well. Look at the covers of the bestselling books in the diet section of any bookstore. The titles imply that we can lose a lot of weight in a ridiculously brief period of time (e.g., days), or that we can eat all the food we want and still lose weight.

As intelligent people we know that neither of these statements is true. It is not physically possible to lose large amounts of weight in very short periods of time, not is it possible to eat more calories than our bodies need and lose weight, no matter what type of food is being eaten. Yet we buy the book hoping against hope that this will be the diet that does the trick once and for all.

It is because of our failures that the diet industry remains so profitable. The business thrives on our inability to stay thin because we then remain eager consumers, once again desperate and willing to try (read: buy) the next miracle cure.

I was one of these people. I wanted the magic that would make me thin forever. In the end, however, it was science, not magic, that came to my rescue.

My Story

In a way, I guess I was lucky. I didn't get heavy until my teen years, escaping the ridicule and torment that elementary school kids usually dole out to their fat classmates. (In retrospect, I hope I wasn't one of the offenders, but I imagine I probably was.)

In high school, no one teased me outright about my appearance, but I suffered nonetheless. My self-esteem was a zero. I hated myself and was consumed with envy; I wanted to be like the other girls, the ones who were thin and attractive. But no matter what diet I tried, and, believe me, I tried them all, I wasn't successful. I *needed* to eat, though I couldn't exactly explain why.

Seeing that my appearance was never going to be my strong point, I figured my best chance of finding success was by developing my intellect. I went to college and majored in psychology. I took a particular interest in behavioral science and behavior therapy, and after two years of study developed a weight-loss program for myself based on these scientific principles. It is still these same principles that form the foundation of my weight-control approach today.

Amazingly, the program worked and within six months I was thin. I mean really thin, from a size 11 down to a size 5. Not only did I lose the weight, I kept it off. Twenty years later, although I'm no longer a junior size, I'm proud to say I am a perfect size 6.

After fifteen years of following this program, I am now making this weight-loss approach available to you. Using this book, in the comfort and privacy of your own home, you will serve as your own therapist. You will learn how to identify, challenge, and change the psychological factors that lead you to overeat. Through this individualized, psychological approach to overeating, you will finally achieve the long-term weight control that has eluded you for so many years.

REPLACING MYTHOLOGY WITH PSYCHOLOGY

The facts are clear—diets don't work. We need an entirely different way of thinking about weight control, one that solves the problem for good rather than supplying a short-term fix.

The psychological approach to treating overeating offers a long-term, permanent solution for weight control. The approach is based on three essential principles, each rooted in behavioral science.

Principle Number 1:
Overeating is a symptom that has psychological causes

You read earlier about the poor long-term outcome for traditional approaches to weight loss. Although reducing our calorie intake will make us and keep us thin, and despite the fact that reduced-calorie products are readily available to us, we aren't able to stay with this approach in the long run.

The eat-less approach to weight loss fails for long-term weight control because it focuses on symptoms rather than focusing on the underlying problems that *cause* the symptoms, which is a Band-Aid method of solving problems. It may provide a short-term fix, but almost never leads to a long-term cure.

If overeating itself is the focus of change, as is the case with virtually all existing weight-loss programs, weight loss will almost always be short-lived. As is the case with any psychological problem, if the symptoms of the problem are treated without addressing their underlying cause, they will, in time, recur.

This accounts for the "yo-yo syndrome," repetitive weight fluctuations, that most chronic dieters experience. Diets, which focus on *what* you eat, will never be effective for long-term weight control because they target the wrong area for change. Overeating continues because its underlying cause has not been addressed.

Professional in the health-care industry are well aware of the importance of identifying and treating the underlying causes of symptoms. Through physical examinations and laboratory tests, they deduce which specific underlying condition is responsible for the presenting symptoms, then prescribe treatment accordingly.

Take the example of a headache, a common physical problem that can have a variety of possible causes. A headache can be a response to stress or a symptom accompanying the flu, can follow a head trauma or concussion, or, in the most extreme circumstances, can result from a tumor or other abnormality in the brain. Because headaches can stem from different causes, and because these different causes necessitate the use of different treatment approaches, it is of major importance to correctly identify which underlying factor is responsible for the symptom.

Imagine that doctors did not proceed in this manner. Suppose they treated all of their patients who complained of headaches in the same way, ignoring the etiology of the symptoms. If this were the case, many people would not respond to treatment—some would continue to experience pain and some, the most severely ill, might actually die.

Overeating, like a headache, is a symptom that reflects an underlying pathology. But in the case of those who are overweight, the pathology usually associated with the condition is psychological.

It is very easy for us to accept the possibility that our excess weight is due to an underlying medical condition. Many of us have hoped that our weight problem was the result of a sluggish metabolism (hypothyroidism) that could easily be corrected with medication. In reality, however, only a very small percentage of overweight people have medical problems that contribute significantly to their weight. For the vast majority of sufferers, it is underlying psychological factors that drive overeating and weight gain.

An interesting example of a physical symptom having a psychological cause can be seen in Charlotte, a fifty-five-year-old married woman who had difficulty walking for fifteen years. Numerous medical examinations and tests were negative and no neurological or other medical cause for her problem was found. As a result, she was referred to me for psychological treatment.

Charlotte had been in a horrendous marriage all of her adult life but was frightened to leave her husband and be on her own. Through working with her, it became clear to me that her inability to walk was very much related to her conflict about her marriage. Her symptoms served an important psychological function: They solved her dilemma about what to do about her marriage, as she now, in her own mind, was unable to leave her husband because she couldn't walk.

In reality, Charlotte's true problem was her feelings of dependency and helplessness, which caused her to remain in an unhealthy marriage. Her problem with walking was simply a symptom, a reflection of and, in some ways, a solution to her psychological conflict (if she couldn't walk, she couldn't leave).

If I had focused on Charlotte's walking and ignored her marital situation, I would have done her a gross injustice and she would not have gotten better. The psychological issues underlying her physical symptom had to be resolved in order for her to be able to walk on her own again.

Overeating and being overweight, while symptoms, reflect psychological problems that must be addressed. Sometimes these problems are complex, as in Charlotte's case, while other times they simply are unproductive behaviors and habits that have been learned and must be unlearned.

It is the variety of psychological causes of overeating that leads us to our next principle.

Principle Number 2:
The psychological causes underlying overeating
are different for different people

Eating when we are not physically hungry is not natural. Wild animals consume food in response to hunger, stopping when they are sated. Similarly, newborn babies take in sustenance only until they have received an adequate amount of nourishment. Likewise, if you observe naturally thin people, you will see that most of them follow the same rule as animals and newborns: Eat when hungry, stop when full.

If eating in the absence of hunger is not a normal behavior, why do so many people do it? Why do people eat when they are not actually, in the true physiological sense of the word, hungry?

Many overeaters point to taste as the reason they overeat—food just tastes too good to resist. In reality, taste plays a fairly small role in the development of overeating. Rather, like many other addictive behaviors, overeating develops because of the physical (neurochemical) and psychological effects this behavior has on us. Eating produces distinct, pleasurable biochemical changes in the body. The physical effects, in turn, have powerful psychological consequences.

In treating overeating, the first line of offense usually is to reduce the amount of food we eat. This strategy, however, never works in the long run, because it ignores the psychological function of overeating in our lives.

The psychological factors that precipitate and perpetuate overeating must be reckoned with if one wants to gain permanent control over one's eating. By addressing the reasons why people overeat, that is, the underlying psychological function of this behavior, the psychological approach to overeating eliminates the true causes of overeating and produces permanent weight control.

What are the psychological factors that lead us to overeat?

Many overeaters use food to decrease the feelings associated with unpleasant emotions. Although this general rule holds true for many, the *particular* negative emotions that fuel overeating are different for everyone.

Some people eat to become happy when they are sad. Others use food to relax when they are tense. Some overweight individuals use food to raise their energy levels when they are tired, while some eat as a diversion when they are bored. Some people use eating as a means to avoid thinking about their problems. Others eat to keep busy when they are ill at ease or self-conscious in social situations. Some use food to try to push or prompt themselves to do things they really don't want to do.

In other words, although many of us strive to change our emotions through eating, the specific negative feelings we frequently feel, and are problematic for our weight, differ.

Take Betty, for instance, who uses food to try to reduce stress and anxiety; when she's tense or uptight she goes to the refrigerator for relief. By contrast, Margaret can't eat at all when she's stressed (her stomach gets queasy) but can't stop eating when she's depressed. And Roberta is like both Betty and Margaret—she overeats in reaction to anxious and depressed feelings.

Betty uses food as a tranquilizer, when she is stressed out, while Margaret uses food as an antidepressant, when she is feeling down, and Roberta uses food for both of these reasons.

Adding to the complexity of the situation, many overeaters have behavioral factors that contribute to their overeating. If we were to make a chart of all the possible combinations of psychological reasons behind overeating, we would see that there are myriad possible overeater profiles or types.

Because people differ in the particular set of emotions and behaviors that cause overeating, the treatment approach to conquering their weight problems also will differ. This leads us to principle number 3.

Principle Number 3:
Permanent weight control is achieved by using psychological treatment methods that directly correspond to the specific causes of overeating for each individual

Since overeating is a symptom that reflects psychological factors that have not been addressed, eating less will not be possible over the long term until we eliminate the psychological causes of this behavior.

To successfully deal with the psychological factors that cause overeating, we need to use psychological treatment methods. What is a psychological treatment? Your immediate response to this term may be to picture a dimly lit office with an older gentleman (perhaps with a beard) sitting behind a desk, pen and paper in hand, and a patient reclining on a sofa facing away from the doctor. While the image in your head would be an accurate reflection of traditional psychoanalytic psychotherapy, it does not depict the types of procedures commonly used by most psychologists today.

The focus in psychological treatment today is on teaching people specific skills that they can use to enhance their lives. Moreover, the techniques themselves must bear up to scientific scrutiny, much the same as for medical treatments.

When I talk about using psychological procedures to treat overeating, I am referring to these self-help techniques. There is no magic or mystery involved with these methods. They are straightforward skills that can be easily understood and learned by almost anyone. The scientific self-help skills to be learned must relate directly to the psychological factors that lead to overeating for a particular person. In other words, the treatment must match the problem. In this way, the treatment approach is individualized.

This orientation is quite different from other weight-loss approaches. Most diets and weight-control programs maintain that their particular approach is the single correct way to combat obesity. The underlying notion here is that all overweight people are overweight for the same reason and that as a result they will respond similarly and successfully to the same, single treatment method. This is simply not the case.

I recently received a telephone call from Harry, a patient whom I had treated nine years earlier. Harry was an anxious overeater. He used food to help him reduce stress and to relax. At the time I first met Harry, he was extremely overweight. In addition to his weight problem, he was having both job and marital difficulties.

Harry and I worked on psychological techniques specifically designed to reduce stress and anxiety. Once he became successful at using these new skills, weight loss followed. Since he no longer needed to use eating as a way to unwind, this unproductive behavior vanished. In addition, because his anxiety had harmful effects on his marriage and employment, he experienced dramatic changes in both of these areas as well.

Today, Harry remains thin, has a great relationship with his wife, and is tremendously successful running his own business. He is an excellent example of the multiple positive effects that can be experienced when the psychological problem underlying overeating rather than overeating itself is treated. His anxiety played a negative role in many areas of his life, including his weight, marriage, and employment. By eliminating the anxiety, all three of these areas improved.

While anxious overeaters like Harry need to conquer their anxiety problems by learning stress-reduction techniques, other treatment approaches are appropriate for other types of overeaters.

Let's look at a few more examples: Nancy was overeating as a way to avoid thinking about her failing marriage. She learned how to confront and solve her marital problems and lost thirty pounds. Susan was using food as entertainment. She discovered how to get enjoyment from other activities and lost twenty-five pounds. Beverly was eating to counter depression. She learned how to improve her mood without food and lost sixty pounds. Matt was using food to avoid thinking about his dead-end job. When he took control of his life and changed his position, he lost twenty pounds. Barbara was snacking to try to boost her energy level. When she addressed her boredom and fatigue head-on, she lost fifteen pounds.

Years later, all of these people are still thin. By identifying the specific psychological problems causing them to overeat and then applying the appropriate psychological treatment methods, they finally succeeded where they had previously failed.

The First Step

In order to enjoy lifelong weight control, you must first give up some long-held beliefs and ideas that stand in your way. You need to stop viewing overeating as the *problem* and begin seeing it as a *symptom* of some other problem. You must cease counting calories and fat grams and be willing to focus on the psychological factors, both emotional and behavioral, that produce overeating. You need to stop measuring your progress by what the scale says (at least for the time being) and instead focus on the development and practice of new skills. By addressing the psychological factors that lead you to overeat, you will lose weight. But more importantly, you will maintain your new weight because you will have permanently eliminated the underlying problems that caused you to overeat.

The program that you are about to embark on is not a diet. There are no special foods to eat, no meal plans to follow, and no recipes to try out. Rather, it contains all of the psychological tools that you need to identify and treat the underlying causes of your weight problem.

You are about to start on a journey that will permanently alter your weight and change your life. Whether you need to lose 10 pounds or 110 pounds, this program will enable you to reach your destination. Like hundreds of others you will experience the joy and freedom that come from conquering destructive behaviors and emotions and gain lifelong control of your weight and your life.

Together we will end the seemingly endless cycle of weight losses and weight gains and turn defeat and despair into victory and exhilaration. The time is now!

1

Identifying the Problem:
How, What, or Why You Eat

When Margie first came to my office she weighed 162 pounds. She wasn't looking for treatment for her weight problem—she believed she had inherited bad genes and would always be overweight. Instead, she wanted to resolve the feelings of sadness that she had experienced on and off since childhood.

After I got to know Margie, it became clear that her bouts with depression were due to a poor self-image. We worked together for about six months, building her self-esteem using a variety of psychological techniques. For the first time in her life, Margie began to feel good about herself and developed an optimistic attitude toward life. Moreover, much to her astonishment, as her sadness dissipated she began to eat less and lose weight.

Why did she lose weight? Because the real cause of her overeating had vanished.

As discussed in the Introduction, while a low-calorie approach to weight loss can help people lose weight, it rarely produces long-term weight control. Diets fail because they focus on the symptom of overeating rather than on the underlying psychological factors that support this type of behavior. When the psychological factors that cause overeating are addressed, the weight comes off and stays off, like it did for Margie.

The psychological factors that cause overeating can be divided into three categories: *how, what,* and *why. How* factors include eating behaviors and habits that encourage overeating (*how* people eat). *What* factors involve food selections (*what* people eat). Finally, *why* factors are the emotional triggers to overeating (*why* people eat).

In order to lose weight, and keep it off, the individual cause of your weight problem must be addressed. If you are overweight because of *why* you eat, focusing on *how* or *what* you eat won't really help you. Similarly, if you overeat because of a problematic eating style—that is, *how* you eat—dealing with *what* or *why* factors will be ineffective.

So let's begin with the first step toward permanent weight control—identifying the how, what, and why causes of your overeating.

YOUR EATING PROFILE

Diagnosis is the procedure commonly used in both medicine and psychology to identify and classify problems. While in medicine there are laboratory and physical tests to arrive at diagnoses, there are no blood tests or X rays for psychological problems. Diagnoses in the mental-health field usually are based on information provided by the person seeking treatment.

To identify and diagnose the psychological factors that cause you to overeat, you need to supply detailed information about your personality traits and eating style. The Eating Profile Questionnaire (EPQ) was designed to help you do this. It explores your personality characteristics and eating behavior. Based on interviews and treatment of hundreds of overweight people, the EPQ was developed to diagnose the five most common causes of overeating. It will provide the data we need to deduce the reasons behind your weight problem.

The questionnaire will take you about ten minutes to complete. Be accurate and honest with your responses—your objective appraisal of yourself is needed in order to make the correct diagnosis and, ultimately, for successful treatment of your weight problem.

The Eating Profile Questionnaire (EPQ)

		Yes	No
1.	Do you often eat standing up?	—	—
2.	Is it difficult for you to remember everything that you ate today or yesterday?	—	—
3.	Do you often eat between meals?	—	—
4.	Do you tend to finish your food before others?	—	—
5.	Do you often not use plates or utensils when eating?	—	—
6.	Do you frequently do other activities while eating?	—	—
7.	Is quality of food more important than quantity?	—	—
8.	Do you tend to eat slowly?	—	—
9.	Do you enjoy trying different types of food?	—	—
10.	Do you love high-fat or high-sugar foods?	—	—
11.	Do you pass on food that isn't tasty?	—	—
12.	Is eating one of your greatest pleasures?	—	—
13.	Are you a nervous or high-strung person?	—	—
14.	Do you often snack when you're tense or uptight?	—	—
15.	Is it hard for you to resist eating something that is right in front of you?	—	—
16.	Is it difficult for you to relax?	—	—
17.	Is the act of eating often more important than what you are eating?	—	—
18.	Are you a worrier?	—	—
19.	Is it difficult for you to be assertive?	—	—
20.	Do you have upsetting dreams?	—	—
21.	Do you often eat to avoid thinking about upsetting things?	—	—
22.	Is it sometimes hard for you to identify your feelings?	—	—
23.	Do you have problems that seem insurmountable?	—	—
24.	Are you a people-pleaser?	—	—
25.	Do you have special feel-good foods?	—	—
26.	Does eating initially give you a lift or a high?	—	—
27.	Do you often feel sad, bored, or down in the dumps?	—	—
28.	Do you often plan out food treats for yourself?	—	—
29.	Are you overly critical of yourself?	—	—
30.	Do you lack energy or enthusiasm?	—	—

Now that you have completed the EPQ, it's time to score it. Using the scoring system below, see which of the five eating profiles apply to you.

Questions 1 through 6: If you answered "yes" to four or more of these questions, you are an Impulse Eater.

Questions 7 through 12: If you answered "yes" to four or more of these questions, you are a Hedonist.

Questions 13 through 18: If you answered "yes" to four or more of these questions, you are a Stress Reducer.

Questions 19 through 24: If you answered "yes" to four or more of these questions, you are an Avoider.

Questions 25 through 30: If you answered "yes" to four or more of these questions, you are an Energizer.

It's a good idea to have another person who knows you well, a spouse, close friend, or relative, complete the EPQ, as if he or she were describing you, to serve as a reality test of your self-perceptions. Sometimes it's hard to see ourselves as we really are; it's difficult to be objective about our shortcomings. If you find there are differences between your answers and those of the other person, give yourself some time to rethink your responses. You may want to observe yourself for a few days, taking notes that relate to the areas covered in the EPQ. Then fill out the questionnaire again, this time using the information gained from your self-observation.

The eating profiles—Impulse Eater, Hedonist, Stress Reducer, Avoider, and Energizer—are shorthand descriptions of the causes of your overeating. While the actual name given to each profile is only a label, it carries a lot of information about your personality and eating behavior.

Now let's see what each category means and how it relates to you.

THE IMPULSE EATER:
TOO BUSY TO PAY ATTENTION TO FOOD

im-pulse: a sudden spontaneous urge to act
—WEBSTER'S DICTIONARY

High-energy and action-oriented people, Impulse Eaters are fun loving and optimistic. They have many interests and cannot tolerate boredom.

Perhaps because they are so busy pursuing life, Impulse Eaters do not pay enough attention to the *act* of eating. They almost always are doing something else while they are eating: talking on the telephone, doing paperwork, watching television. Because they are in a hurry, they grab food that's fast or looks good without thinking of the consequences. They eat quickly, without concentrating on the taste or texture of the food.

Because of their style of eating, Impulse Eaters end up consuming too many calories by eating too much food, and gain weight.

Let's take a look at some real-life examples:

Ann is forty years old and has been overweight for most of her adult life. She is an overachiever and spends most of her time at the office or on her many projects. She's always on the move and rarely takes time to sit back and relax.

Although overall she is a happy person, Ann has one area in her life that causes her distress: her weight. She started to put on extra pounds in college and has continued to gain weight ever since. During the last few years she has been carrying around an extra forty-five pounds. Although she has lost weight a number of times, she never has been able to keep it off for more than a few months.

When I first met Ann, she expressed confusion about her excess weight: "I really don't eat a lot...I don't know why I weigh so much!"

Ann completed the EPQ and it was clear why she is overweight: She is an Impulse Eater.

Ann has some very bad eating habits. She often eats on the run, either in her car, while working on a project in her office, or in between meals. She is an extremely fast eater, always being the first one to finish a meal. She frequently eats while standing up, not using a plate, knife, or fork. She snacks incessantly and is not particularly fussy about what she eats.

Because she is not paying attention to the act of eating, Ann has trouble remembering exactly what she consumes on any given day. When I asked her what she had eaten for breakfast that morning, she told me scrambled eggs and orange juice. It was only by asking her husband the same question that I learned Ann also had three leftover strips of bacon and two pieces of buttered toast from her kids' plates.

Ann is unaware of all she is eating because food does not play a lead role in her life. While at first this may sound like it wouldn't cause a weight problem, let's take a look at the facts.

Ann has no set mealtime. She eats whenever she can fit it into her busy schedule and does so quickly, without concern for the quality of the food. Because eating is not a memorable occasion, she has trouble recalling exactly what she had to eat, even on that very day.

Like Ann, Dee, a young stay-at-home mother with two toddlers, is also eating on a catch-as-catch-can basis. Most of her eating is done standing in front of an open refrigerator door. She finishes whatever leftovers are on the kids' plates as well as eating "grown-up" meals with her husband. Given how active she is with her two youngsters, she can't understand why she is overweight.

Ann and Dee are both experiencing the same problem. Their eating habits are causing them to overeat and gain weight. The Impulse Eater shows the following characteristics:

- Eats quickly
- Eats on the run
- Engages in other activities while eating
- Has trouble remembering everything that was eaten
- Eats in "noneating" places (on sofa, in car, standing up)
- Snacks a lot
- Eats with hands (no plate, fork, knife)
- Is not particular about type of food

Despite their weight problems, Impulse Eaters tend to be happy people. They are active, usually intense, and enjoy the things they do. They are goal-directed individuals who make the most out of life.

If you are an Impulse Eater you're in good company. It is one of the most common reasons for being overweight and is shared by millions of men and women.

The good news is that impulse eating is easy to fix. With the right techniques and practice, Impulse Eaters change their eating style readily. Once they do this, they shed the fat and take delight in their new, thin selves.

Impulse Eaters are overweight because of how they eat—their eating style.

Now let's turn to the Hedonist, who has an entirely different problem.

THE HEDONIST: EATING FOR PLEASURE

he-do-nism: a doctrine that pleasure is the chief good in life
—WEBSTER'S DICTIONARY

Hedonists are outgoing, adventurous people. They are always looking for a good time and they usually find it. They experience the joys of life to the fullest, and take the time to smell the roses.

For Hedonists, the pursuit of pleasure extends to their eating. They derive immense satisfaction from their food, paying close attention to the texture, smell, and taste of everything they eat. Eating is an important experience that is done slowly and given complete attention.

Because they are pleasure eaters, Hedonists consume too many calories and gain weight. Their problem is their food selections.

Here are two actual cases from my practice:

Susan loves to eat. She gets tremendous enjoyment from food and considers mealtime to be an important event. She remembers every morsel that she eats, easily recalling favorite meals from the past, and spends a lot of time talking about them.

As opposed to the Impulse Eater, Susan always sits down when eating, eats slowly, and uses the appropriate utensils. She never eats on the run or in front of the refrigerator.

An amateur gourmet chef, Susan's favorite hobby is cooking. She enjoys experimenting with different recipes and particularly loves developing new sauces for entrées. She frequently entertains at home but also likes to dine out. She is adventurous in her eating and will try almost any food at least once. However, if a food does not appeal to her, she turns up her nose at it.

Susan is carrying around an extra twenty-five pounds because she is a Hedonist. Her score on the EPQ shows that the source of her being overweight is pleasure eating. Food plays too great a role in Susan's life. Susan lives to eat instead of eating to live. Rather than assuming an appropriate place in her life, eating *is* Susan's life. Although she has good eating habits—sitting down when eating, not snacking much, eating slowly—her preoccupation with food is doing her in.

Darlene, like Susan, also is a Hedonist. At sixty, her children are grown and her husband is retired. Not a cook herself, she and her husband eat out most nights. Darlene loves to try new restaurants and is particularly fond of those that offer several courses for a fixed price. Desserts, especially chocolate ones, are her greatest passion. Despite the fact that she is an avid tennis player and exercises at a health club five days a week, Darlene is thirty pounds overweight.

Susan and Darlene both are heavy because of their food selections: what they eat. They are drawn to high-calorie foods because of their taste appeal and ability to generate pleasure. The Hedonist has the following traits:

- Eats slowly
- Looks forward to mealtimes
- Remembers exactly what was eaten
- Likes to talk about food
- Chooses quality of food over quantity
- Passes on food that isn't tasty
- Loves to cook or dine out
- Consumes a lot of high-fat or high-sugar foods

Even though they are concerned about their weight, Hedonists generally are very happy and fun people. They are optimistic and enthusiastic, eager to try new things and go to new places.

If you are a Hedonist, don't be overly concerned—most people take pleasure in eating. But to lose weight and stay thin, Hedonists must make some changes in what they eat and develop a new perspective toward food. Once they do this the weight comes off and stays off!

Hedonists are overweight because of what they eat—high-calorie foods.

The next three types of overeaters, the Stress Reducer, the Avoider, and the Energizer, all have why factors leading to overeating. However, the particular situations and emotions that cause overeating are different for each.

THE STRESS REDUCER: USING FOOD TO UNWIND

stress: a factor that induces bodily or mental tension
—WEBSTER'S DICTIONARY

Stress Reducers are sensitive and imaginative human beings. They have tremendous drive, and when they channel their energies to meet their goals they are enormously productive and successful.

Unfortunately, the pent-up feelings that lead them to great accomplishments are the same feelings that cause them to overeat. Stress Reducers have gotten into a bad habit of using food to reduce tension. By eating in response to stress and using food to unwind, Stress Reducers overeat and get heavy.

Sherry is a nervous and emotional young woman. Although things are going well in her life—her commercial-art business is flourishing and she is engaged to be married to a wonderful young man—Sherry is on edge most of the time and has difficulty relaxing.

Sherry has always been high strung. Even as an infant, her mother remembers her as being colicky. As a young girl, she was fearful of new situations such as her first haircut, beginning school, and sleeping over at other children's homes. As she got older she developed new anxieties about herself, about her relationships with others, and about work.

Sherry has a lot of nervous habits. She plays with her hair, bites her fingernails, and has trouble sitting still. Her mind is always going, worrying about the past, the present, and the future. She is a worrywart.

When Sherry eats she has trouble stopping. The idea of being full is foreign to her; she doesn't know what it means. She's more involved with the activities of eating—chewing and swallowing—than with the effect on her stomach. When I met Sherry for the first time, she confided that she feels out of control: "It's like I'm compulsive or something...I just can't seem to stop eating."

As her score on the EPQ indicates, Sherry is using food to reduce stress and to relax. She is a Stress Reducer. Her worries and fears lead her to the refrigerator and, once there, she can't stop eating. Sherry uses food as someone else might use a sedative or tranquilizer. She attempts to eliminate the symptoms of anxiety, the worries, the fears, the tension in her body, by eating.

Phil, a real-estate investor, has a lot in common with Sherry. A recovering alcoholic, he has been using food to relax ever since he gave up drinking. On workdays, Phil frequently visits the vending machine down the hall from his office for snacks. At night, in an attempt to unwind, he eats in front of the television.

The Stress Reducer, like Sherry and Phil, exhibits these behaviors:

- Is nervous or high strung
- Worries a lot
- Has trouble relaxing
- Eats quickly
- Tends to be fearful
- Frequently eats in "noneating" places (in front of the refrigerator)
- Eats more as stress increases

In addition to being overeaters, some Stress Reducers have problems with alcohol or cigarettes. They use these substances as well as food to calm their nerves. Interestingly, because their eating is related to stress, Stress Reducers often lose weight when on vacation, when they are away from the pressures of everyday life.

Creative and energetic, Stress Reducers have the capacity for great accomplishments. When they put their energies toward a project they are tremendously successful. Because of these traits, motivated Stress Reducers cannot be stopped from achieving their goals. If you fit this profile, and your goal is permanent weight control, there is no doubt you will get there. Learning how to eliminate anxiety without eating will get you where you want to be.

Stress Reducers are overweight because of why they eat—to eliminate anxiety.

The next type of overeater, the Avoider, is also overweight because of emotional triggers. However, in this case, the triggers are not as easy to observe.

THE AVOIDER: ESCAPING LIFE'S PROBLEMS WITH FOOD

avoid: to keep away from; shun
—WEBSTER'S DICTIONARY

Avoiders are warm and compassionate people. They are sensitive to other people's feelings and would not hurt a fly. They have lifelong friends who can count on them for almost anything.

Although Avoiders are great at listening to and helping others, they have a hard time dealing with their own problems. Instead of confronting and solving their difficulties, they try to forget about them with food. Avoiders overeat to escape dealing with life's problems. This is why they are overweight.

Let's look at two real-life examples:

Phyllis is in a bad marriage. Her husband has been cheating on her for years. She has stayed with him for the sake of the children, but now that the kids are grown and out of the house she really can't justify remaining in the marriage.

Phyllis has always been somewhat timid. It is very difficult for her to speak her mind for fear that she might hurt or upset another person. She puts other people's needs in front of her own, and hasn't given much thought to who she is or what she wants out of life.

Despite her problems, Phyllis has a lot of friends, interests, and hobbies. She has filled the void created by an absentee husband with other pursuits.

Many nights Phyllis is awakened by terrible dreams. When she wakes up she immediately heads to the kitchen for something to eat, trying to get the dreams out of her head. These frequent trips to the refrigerator have caused her to put on quite a bit of weight.

At our first meeting Phyllis told me that her attitude toward problems is to ignore them and they will go away. However, so far the problems have not gone away and while she is waiting for them to disappear, she's having nightmares and overeating. Her EPQ score shows that she is an Avoider.

Phyllis overeats to avoid facing life's problems. Rather than solving her problems, she passively waits for something to change while suppressing her thoughts and feelings with food.

Janet is also an Avoider. A college professor, she is unhappy with her job. She is making a good salary and has excellent benefits, but the job no longer holds interest for her as she's been teaching the same courses for years. Because of the job's salary and benefits she is having a difficult time justifying leaving her position. She occasionally has thoughts of trying something new but immediately pushes them out of her head. The idea of change is too overwhelming.

Janet, like Phyllis, has been overweight for years. Instead of solving her problem, she pushes it away with food.

The Avoider has the following profile:

- Has trouble identifying feelings
- Has difficulty being assertive
- Puts the needs of others first
- Ignores problems, hoping they will go away
- Has upsetting dreams
- Eats to avoid thinking about problems
- Eats more as problems worsen
- Eats in "noneating" places (on sofa, standing up)

Most Avoiders are women. Although it is not clear whether this is due to genetic predisposition, environment, upbringing, or a combination of these factors, women are more likely than men to be passive in the face of difficulties and to put the desires of other people before their own.

In an attempt to suppress their thoughts and feelings, Avoiders, like Stress Reducers, may turn to alcohol.

Although Avoiders, like all people, have their shortcomings, they also possess many strengths. Avoiders are often caring and sensitive people who have great concern for others. They are typically very loyal friends who would give you the shirt off their backs.

If you are an Avoider, you can learn to confront and solve your problems. Although it will take some work, the payoff is tremendous. Not only will you take control of your weight, you will take control of your entire life.

Avoiders are overweight because of why they eat—to escape dealing with their problems.

The last type of overeater is the Energizer. Let's see which emotion is the problem here.

THE ENERGIZER: USING FOOD AS A PICK-ME-UP

en-er-gize: to strengthen body or mind in order to do things
—WEBSTER'S DICTIONARY

Energizers are bright, thinking people who look at things at the deepest level. They tend to be serious about the things they do, usually showing precision and attention to detail.

Maybe because of their depth and perfectionism, Energizers can easily become dissatisfied. They often feel sad, bored, or tired. When they feel this way, they use food as a pick-me-up.

By eating to feel better, Energizers consume too much and gain weight.

Let's take a look at these examples:

Rhonda is unhappy. For most of her adult life she's been troubled by sadness and feelings of emptiness. Depression runs in her family, and she assumes there is nothing she can do about it.

Although she is successful in her own business, Rhonda sees herself as a failure. She is extremely critical of herself and thinks that other people don't like her. She is tired much of the time and lacks enthusiasm.

Rhonda eats to get a lift. She feels good while she's eating, but soon after feels even worse than before, guilty and full of self-hatred. Her attempt to improve her mood through food has the opposite effect and she ends up even more depressed.

Rhonda knows why she is heavy. Her score on the EPQ confirms what she already suspected, that she is an Energizer. "I know I eat to feel better and it doesn't work... I just don't know how to break out of this."

Rhonda uses food as an antidepressant. She's caught in a vicious cycle: feeling bad, overeating to counter the bad feelings, feeling worse, eating again to feel better, and so on.

Margaret also is an Energizer but, unlike Rhonda, she doesn't know it. She does not have feelings of sadness though she frequently feels bored. She has no hobbies or interests. She is a loner and doesn't spend much time with other people. She says, "Food is my best friend."

Unfortunately, Margaret's best friend is ruining her life. She is morbidly obese, weighing 280 pounds, and has many weight-related health problems.

The Energizer has these characteristics:

- Is often sad, bored, or tired
- Tries to get a lift from food
- Suffers from low self-esteem
- Plans food treats
- Feels depressed after eating
- Considers food to be a best friend
- Has a pessimistic view of the future

Because Energizers are self-critical and lack self-esteem, they often are socially anxious. Being uncomfortable around other people, they are at risk of overeating in social situations.

Of all the types of overeaters, Energizers are the most likely to see their weight problem as hopeless. This stems from their negative outlook on life and does not reflect their actual likelihood of success.

Like Stress Reducers and Avoiders, Energizers may abuse alcohol. Although alcohol actually is a depressant, Energizers use it to try to raise their moods.

Energizers are typically intelligent people, often interesting conversationalists who have thought-provoking ideas. When they start to feel better about themselves, they focus more on the outside world and less on their own thoughts and feelings.

If you are an Energizer you are not alone. Millions of people battle the same feelings you do. By using the correct methods for your problem, you will eliminate the pain and start experiencing the pleasure that life has to offer. As you feel increased energy and vitality, your eating and weight will decrease.

Energizers are overweight because of why they eat—to improve their moods.

You now should have a good understanding of the five types of overeaters. Just to be sure, take a look at the Problem Identification chart below, which summarizes the primary causes of overeating for each of the five eating profiles.

Problem Identification

Problem	Impulse Eater	Hedonist	Stress Reducer	Avoider	Energizer
How:					
Eating style	X				
What:					
Food selections		X			
Why:					
Reduce anxiety			X		
Escape problems				X	
Lift mood					X

WHAT IF I HAVE MORE THAN ONE PROFILE?

The case histories described in this chapter each highlight only one type of eating profile. However, it is important for you to understand that most overweight people fit into more than one category. In fact, I treated one woman who had the characteristics of all five profiles.

The number of profiles that describe you does not determine your likelihood of success. Whether you meet criteria for two, three, or even all five of the categories, you have the same opportunity as anyone else to permanently conquer your weight problem.

Just as the number of categories that fit your overeating is unrelated to your success, so are the specific types of categories. Whether you are a how, what, or why eater, using the treatment techniques that relate directly to the causes of your weight problem will enable you to lose the weight and keep it off for the years to come.

THE PROGRAM

Now that you have identified the reasons behind your overeating, you are ready to proceed to the heart of this book: the treatment program. Chapters 2 through 6 contain the psychological treatment methods that will eliminate the problematic behaviors and emotions that are responsible for your excess weight.

It is essential that you read all of the chapters that apply to you, that is, those that deal with your overeating profiles. However it is also a very good idea to read *all* of the treatment chapters. Although you may not show all of the signs of a particular profile, you probably have some of the features. You will benefit from using many of the psychological exercises or "psychercises" included for that profile.

The questionnaires, checklists, and written assignments that appear in the treatment chapters have been carefully designed to help you build the skills you need to overcome your weight problem. Do not skip these! They are a necessary part of the treatment program and will help you develop the tools to achieve your goal.

While you are learning the psychological techniques during the course of this program, do not weigh yourself! I know that for most of you this will be very difficult. However, it is *essential* that you refrain from weighing yourself until you have mastered the techniques and eliminated the psychological causes of your overeating. Since your weight loss will begin after you have completed the program, checking your weight before this time is not productive.

I promise that after you have fully developed these techniques you will lose weight! Then you can periodically weigh yourself (no more than once a week, please) to note your progress.

Regardless of which type (or types) of overeating applies to you, it is very important that you reward yourself for learning and practicing your new psychological skills. Rewards can include praising yourself, going to a particular place or event, buying yourself something special, but not eating. *Never use food as a reward!*

You can give yourself small rewards on a daily basis (like renting a videotape movie that you have been wanting to see), larger rewards on a weekly basis (like having a manicure or buying that new bestselling book), and big rewards (like tickets to the theater or a new dress) for completing each month of the program. Be generous in rewarding yourself—you deserve it!

2

The Impulse Eater:
Getting Your Act Together

Sara doesn't understand why she has a weight problem. She is very active and energetic, so she should be burning a lot of calories. She thinks the problem must be something physical, but her physician hasn't found a medical reason for her being overweight.

As a last resort, Sara came to see me. I asked her about her eating habits—how frequently she eats, where she has her meals, if she eats slowly or on the run. She had a hard time answering my questions, so I suggested she keep a daily record of her eating behavior until our next session.

After a week of keeping her log, Sara was shocked to see how often she was eating: an average of once an hour. Keeping a record forced her to pay attention to what and when she was eating. Identifying this problem behavior was Sara's first step toward gaining control of her weight once and for all.

As you read in chapter 1, Impulse Eaters are overweight because of bad eating behaviors. How food is eaten, rather than what kind of food or why food is eaten, is the primary cause of weight gain for this group of overeaters.

Impulse Eaters do not pay enough attention to the *act* of eating, often eating on the run or standing up, not using utensils, and not having set mealtimes. Because they do not pay enough attention to the act of eating, they eat a larger quantity of food and eat too often.

My husband is an excellent example of an Impulse Eater. He has been fifteen pounds overweight since the day I met him and is not really interested in losing the weight. However, if he wanted to drop the pounds and keep them off he would need to make some major changes in his behavior.

Like most Impulse Eaters, my husband cannot accurately recall what he has eaten on any given day. That's because he does not pay attention to his eating—he does most of his eating standing up in the kitchen. Moreover, he often does not use a plate. He eats very quickly, takes large bites, and doesn't pay attention to the taste or texture of his food. He gobbles rather than savors.

Because of his inattentive eating behavior, he thinks he's hungry much more often than is actually possible. Quite frankly, I'm not sure he has ever gone long enough without food to know what hunger really feels like.

Compare my eating behavior to his: I always sit down at the kitchen table when I eat, always use a plate and utensils when appropriate, and eat slowly, taking small bites, savoring each and every morsel of food. As a result of my attentive eating behaviors, I only eat when I am hungry, and I almost never overeat.

I didn't always have such good eating habits. I used to be a lot like my husband. But by applying psychological techniques to my eating behavior, I was able to develop new, positive eating habits.

If you are an Impulse Eater, you can do the same. You can change your eating behavior by following this program. By focusing on how you eat, you will be getting to the root cause of your weight problem.

THE CAUSES OF INATTENTIVE, IMPULSIVE EATING

To some extent, inattentive, impulsive eating styles are a by-product of living in this country. The fact that fast-food eating originated here in the United States is a testimony to this.

Doing things quickly, and doing several things at once, is an American tradition. We eat breakfast in our car on our way to work, saving the time of sitting down to have breakfast at home. If we do allow ourselves the luxury of eating breakfast at home, it's usually something microwavable or easily prepared that can also be eaten quickly.

It is not unusual to eat lunch in our office while doing paperwork or handling phone calls. If we do go out for lunch, we typically drive to the nearest fast-food restaurant, possibly ordering from, and then eating inside, our car. If we are at home caring for children, we often eat what's left on their plates rather than sitting down for our own meal.

Dinner, the main meal of the day for most families, also is eaten haphazardly; with Dad coming home late from a business meeting, Johnny having an after-school soccer match, and Mary's Girl Scout troop coming over to the house, everyone is eating dinner at different times and on the run.

Given the relatively low priority we afford to mealtimes, is it any wonder that much of our population are becoming inattentive and impulsive eaters?

Look at other cultures that place a greater value on mealtimes. In most European, South American, and Asian cultures, the concept of fast food and fast eating is far less prevalent than in the United States (the prevalence of obesity is also substantially less).

The French are known for their long dinners; you don't see them eating a Big Mac in their cars. In England, breakfast together is a family tradition. Although we may take issue with the high-fat content of some of the more popular foods included in a traditional English breakfast, ample time and attention are given to this first meal of the day.

In many countries with a warmer climate, lunch is the primary meal of the day. Sufficient time is delegated from the workday for a leisurely noontime meal, followed by a nap or *siesta,* then a return to work until the early evening hours.

In these countries meals are important events and are given enough time and attention to enjoy them. Eating is planned, not impulsive, and serious weight problems are far less common. By defining set mealtimes, unnecessary eating between meals is reduced.

This is not to say that culture is the only factor contributing to inattentive, impulsive eating. Temperament and personality type also play a role. Hyperactive, Type-A individuals are more likely to develop an impulsive eating style than mellow and relaxed Type-B individuals. Type-A people by definition are intense, goal oriented, and fast moving. These characteristics are at odds with the concept of slow, leisurely dining. By contrast, Type-B adults, who by nature tend to smell the roses, are generally quite comfortable with the idea of devoting time and attention to meals.

Lifestyle also can play a major role in people's eating behaviors. Take the example of a young woman working a full-time job and raising three small children on her own. Slow leisurely meals are a luxury that a woman like this very rarely gets to enjoy.

Whether you have developed an inattentive and impulsive eating style because of personal characteristics, because of your current lifestyle, or simply because you live in a fast-food society, you can learn to change your eating habits. Focusing on *how* you eat, rather than the more traditional approach of focusing on what you eat, will get you, as an Impulse Eater, where you want to go.

THE PSYCHOLOGICAL APPROACH TO IMPULSIVE OVEREATING

The Program for the Impulse Eater contains the specific treatment methods that eliminate this type of overeating. The list includes four different procedures, all of which are designed to get rid of problematic eating behaviors.

In order to become more attentive to and less impulsive in your eating, you must learn how to change both your eating environment and your eating style. You also will learn how to use positive reinforcement techniques (rewards and self-praise) to help develop your new eating behaviors and aversive imagery to suppress your old eating behaviors.

Program for the Impulse Eater

Treatment Method	Begin
Changing your eating environment	Week 1
Positive reinforcement for increasing appropriate eating	Week 2
Changing your eating style	Week 3
Aversive imagery for reducing inappropriate eating	Week 4

Before you get started on this program, it is important that you keep a detailed record of your eating behavior for at least a week. By monitoring your eating behavior you will learn where your areas of weakness lie. Keeping track of your eating will also help you begin to pay more attention to the *act* of eating, something Impulse Eaters are notoriously bad at.

In fact, it is possible that the self-monitoring by itself will produce positive changes in your eating behavior. Research has shown that self-monitoring often has a "reactive effect," that is, it induces positive change on its own (this is thought to occur as a consequence of devoting more attention to whatever problem you are monitoring).

Create a Daily Food Log as the one below and complete it every day for at least a week. Keep the record close at hand at all times so that you can list everything that you eat each day. Even a single hard candy needs to be accounted for.

Daily Food Log

Food		Situation			
Type	Quantity	Where	When	With Whom	Meal?
Example:					
Oreos	4	Office	3 P.M.	Alone	No

Once you have recorded at least seven days' worth of food intake, take a look at your log and see if any patterns emerge.

Are you doing a lot of eating in between meals? Do you do a lot of your eating when you are in the company of a certain person or persons? Do you tend to eat at a particular place or time of the day? Does a particular type of food keep reappearing in your log? Is eating large amounts of food a recurring problem?

Your food log gives you clues about your particular problem areas. For some people certain types of foods seem to encourage overeating. For others the time of day or whom they are with is a more important determinant of overeating.

Keep this information about yourself in mind as you begin to work on changing your eating environment.

CHANGING YOUR EATING ENVIRONMENT

Your environment plays a powerful role in your eating. The physical features of your surroundings, where you are, who you are with, what time of day it is, what you are doing, can cue you into eating, even when you are not hungry.

Perhaps the most obvious example of how your environment triggers you into eating is when you are around other people who are eating. How many times have you been at a social gathering where you continue to eat because other people are eating, despite the fact that you are not hungry? Or how about watching television and a commercial pops up showing an actor consuming a mouthwatering treat? Do you get off of the couch and head for the refrigerator?

While what you see greatly influences what you eat, other aspects of your environment are equally likely to trigger you into unnecessary eating.

In this section we discuss the specific ways in which you can modify your surroundings to reduce the likelihood of overeating. By making these changes you will be controlling your eating environment and, consequently, controlling your eating behavior.

Environmental Change Number 1: Limit Where You Eat

Many of us are in the habit of eating wherever the mood strikes us. We eat in our cars, in movie theaters, malls, restaurants, while walking on the street, in many places besides our homes. Even in our homes we eat in rooms not designed for eating, in family rooms, bedrooms, living rooms.

Because Impulse Eaters do not pay enough attention to the act of eating, they need to make eating more of an occasion, rather than something that happens frequently and without any fanfare. By limiting locations and places where eating takes place, you can exert more control over your eating. You will narrow the opportunities for eating by making rules about where eating can occur.

The first step is to designate one location in your home as the place where you will do your eating. For most people, this will be at the kitchen or dining room table. What this means is that from now on the only place in your home where you will consume food will be when you are seated at your kitchen table. No more snacking on the family room sofa, no midnight cookies and milk in your bedroom, no taste testing as you cook, and no eating standing up. From this point forward, all eating at home will take place in one location only, with no exceptions.

Limiting your eating to one place will probably be more difficult than you expect. As an Impulse Eater, you are used to eating wherever the urge hits you. Most of the time, Impulse Eaters aren't even aware that they are eating; the behavior has become so habitual that it is not even noticed.

You need to begin to pay attention to your eating. By limiting where you allow eating to occur, you will decrease the frequency of unnecessary eating and increase the amount of attention you pay to necessary eating.

The concept is not all that dissimilar from the training you received as a child. As a young child you gained control over your bladder and bowel functions by learning to discriminate between appropriate and inappropriate places to relieve yourself. Through making these discriminations you obtained control over your elimination habits.

Now as an adult, you will gain control over your eating by discriminating between appropriate and inappropriate places to eat. By narrowing down your choices, you will narrow the opportunities for eating and consequently decrease the likelihood that inappropriate eating, or overeating, will occur.

That takes care of while you are at home, but what about eating outside of home and in restaurants, at the office, while traveling? The answer to this is simple but one you probably won't like: *Don't eat outside of your home unless absolutely necessary!*

Some situations will be easier to eliminate than others. It probably won't be all that difficult to cut out eating in your car, at the movie theater, at the food court at the mall, and at the vending machine in your office building. On the other hand, I realize there are important social activities that often include eating away from home such as parties and holiday gatherings. Obviously, you don't want to miss these events. But there are many times when eating away from home is not essential and can be eliminated with a little forethought.

For instance, for many people the weekend includes Saturday night out for dinner with a spouse and/or friends. In this context, eating is a form of entertainment, setting the occasion for interacting with other people.

But aren't there many other ways that you can interact with the important people in your life that are entertaining and do not include eating? Would it be possible for you to suggest an alternative to dining in a restaurant for next Saturday? Maybe a movie without the Chinese food afterward, or bowling without the pizza beforehand?

Try to substitute activities other than eating as forms of entertainment as much as possible. You may be surprised to find that the other individuals in your life welcome the change as well (remember, eating out also is expensive).

Environmental Change Number 2: Limit When You Eat

Just as it is important to limit the places where eating will occur, it is also as important to limit the times of the day when this behavior will take place.

Impulse Eaters, for the most part, are used to eating whenever they feel like it, without regard to whether or not they are actually hungry. Since eating happens without thinking, any time is considered an acceptable time to eat.

To get control over your eating, you must narrow the times of day that are permissible for eating. By deliberately decreasing the occasions for consuming food, your present free-for-all approach to eating will be transformed into attentive, controlled, *intentional* behavior. You will now be in control of your eating, rather than your eating being in control of you.

When should you schedule your eating? Obviously you need to set aside at least three mealtimes that work well with your daily schedule. Since you now are going to be eating at home as much as possible, this should also influence the times of day you choose for your meals. If you work outside of the home, try to have breakfast and dinner at home, and designate a set time to have lunch during your work hours.

Another consideration is to space your meals so that your body does not suffer from low blood sugar. Generally speaking, leaving no more than four or five hours between meals should help you to avoid this problem.

Some people prefer to eat more frequent but smaller meals. This is fine as long as the meals are scheduled and do not occur on impulse.

By only eating during preset times, you will no longer be eating whenever the mood strikes you. Just like discriminating between appropriate and inappropriate places to eat, you will be distinguishing between appropriate and inappropriate times to eat. Limiting the opportunities for eating will help you get rid of the impulsive eating that is at the core of your weight problem.

Environmental Change Number 3: Limit What You Eat

If you don't have it you can't eat it!

As an Impulse Eater you are tempted to eat what's available. Making problem foods less accessible will greatly reduce your consumption of them.

Impulse Eaters tend to be somewhat lazy in their eating. By this I mean that if a food is not readily available, they are unlikely to go out of their way to get it. (This is in opposition to the Hedonist in chapter 3 who will go to great lengths to get his or her hands on a tasty treat.) Therefore, by keeping problem foods out of your home, you will be helping yourself immensely.

Keep problem foods out of your home simply by not buying them! One way to do this is to shop at the supermarket from a list you have made up beforehand, only buying foods that are on your list. As an aside, never go grocery shopping when you are hungry. You will be much more likely to cave in and buy foods that are not on your list on an empty stomach than on a full stomach.

If you must have problem foods in your home because of the others you live with such as your roommate, spouse, or children, keep the goodies out of sight and out of reach. For Impulse Eaters, seeing usually ends up becoming eating; visual cues are highly salient ones that trigger eating for you. You can decrease the likelihood of eating a problem food that is in your home by placing it out of sight or covering it with an opaque wrap like aluminum foil so that you can't see it.

Make problem food that is in the home harder to get to. Put it on a high shelf that requires a stepstool to reach or, if possible, freeze the item. For Impulse Eaters, food that is not right there, ready to eat, is also much less likely to be consumed.

Do not serve meals family style. Sitting at the table with platters of food in front of you is an invitation to an eating disaster. Remember, for the Impulse Eater, seeing is eating and it is far better to keep the food on the kitchen counter and have each family member take his or her own servings from there.

Finally, leave the table as soon as you are finished with your meal. Continuing to sit at the kitchen table watching others eat will only serve as a trigger to eat even though you are no longer hungry. Also, since the kitchen table is now your stimulus for eating, simply being in this location will be a strong trigger for eating.

If you cannot leave the situation, at least remove your plate from the table to discourage continued eating; but it is best to leave the situation altogether when you are finished.

THE POWER OF POSITIVE REINFORCEMENT

All animals, from a single-cell amoeba to a human infant, respond to positive reinforcement. The very definition of positive reinforcement is based on the fact that it works: *Positive reinforcement is the application of something following a behavior that increases the likelihood that that behavior will recur.* In simpler terms, if you reward an activity, its frequency increases.

The something that is applied as a reward can be a tangible item, an event, or verbal praise by yourself or by others. Let's start by discussing the benefits of tangible rewards.

Although we may not think of it as such, we make frequent use of tangible rewards in our daily life. You allow your children to go out and play after they finish their homework. You reward your spouse with a favorite meal for cleaning out the garage. You plan a vacation after completing a special project at work. You buy yourself new clothes when you get a promotion.

Rewards, or positive reinforcement, have tremendous power to change behavior. We can harness that power by learning how to use it systematically to build and strengthen new habits. For Impulse Eaters, that means using it to develop and maintain new eating behaviors.

But what constitutes a positive reinforcer? This is a very individual matter, as what is rewarding for one person is not rewarding to another. What might be a very effective positive reinforcer for me may be totally ineffective for you.

Some people find certain material objects to be highly rewarding. A new outfit, a special collection of compact discs, or redecorating the master bedroom can effectively motivate them. Others respond better to events or activities like going to a concert, having a manicure, or a romantic evening alone at home with their spouse.

In order for rewards to work they must be rewarding to you. Therefore, before you can learn how to use them to your benefit, you need to come up with a list of reinforcements that will be effective for you. You will need small rewards that are easy and inexpensive and that you can use on a daily basis, as well as larger rewards that are more costly or more complicated and that you can use weekly or monthly.

Use the form below to develop your list of positive reinforcements.

Positive Reinforcements

Small Rewards:

1. _____

2. _____

3. _____

4. _____

5. _____

Large Rewards:

1. _____

2. _____

3. _____

4. _____

5. _____

Once you have a list of rewards, we can talk about how best to use them. In the previous section of this chapter, I outlined three environmental changes that will help you decrease your inattentive and impulsive eating. The first change involves restricting the locations where you eat, the second limits the times of day when you eat, and the third limits your access to food.

Although these changes don't sound all that difficult at first, turning them into new habits, new patterns of behavior that are followed consistently, takes some work. Rewards, because they increase the frequency of desired behaviors, are very helpful when trying to establish new habits like these.

As you are changing these behaviors, use your small rewards as daily reinforcements. You might think that rewarding yourself for following the program for one day is overdoing it a bit, but when you are first trying to establish a new habit it is very important to reward yourself frequently and immediately for positive changes. Later on, once the new behavior is more firmly implanted, you can up the ante by requiring more days of success from yourself before receiving a reward.

Although tangible rewards are very effective for changing behavior, there is another type of positive reinforcement that also is effective, and much easier and less costly to administer—praise. It takes only seconds to tell yourself that you have done a good job.

Try to reward your behavior changes not only with tangible items but with self-praise as well. In the early stages of changing your eating environment, try to praise yourself repeatedly during the course of the day as you successfully make changes. This will help motivate you to continue your pattern of success throughout the rest of the day.

You also can ask others who live with you to praise you for making behavior changes. However, make sure that you give them specific guidelines as to what you are supposed to be doing so that they don't end up praising you for the wrong thing.

Two final notes of caution. First, *never* use food as a reward. For obvious reasons, it is extremely counterproductive for anyone with a weight problem to use food as a positive reinforcement. (This is akin to having an alcoholic reinforce alcohol abstinence with a drink!)

Second, remember to reward behavior change, *not* weight change. Although changing your eating behaviors will result in weight loss, it is these new eating habits, not the weight loss, that need to be the target of your reinforcement efforts. If you reward weight loss instead of behavior change, you cannot be sure exactly which behavior you are reinforcing. There are, after all, a lot of things that can result in your losing weight such as increased exercise, lower calorie consumption, having the flu, or using laxatives.

Since making the behavior changes outlined in this program is the only way for Impulse Eaters to gain permanent control over their weight, you must be sure that you are rewarding these changes and not other, irrelevant ones.

SLOW DOWN, YOU MOVE TOO FAST

To get thin and stay thin, Impulse Eaters must not only change their eating environment, but also change how they go about the task of eating, their eating style.

The eating style of the Impulse Eater is inattentive and fast. By slowing down and paying more attention to the act of eating, Impulse Eaters consume less food, and consequently lose weight.

Just as when working on changing your eating environment, use your positive reinforcements to help make changes in your eating style. Remember, start with small daily rewards while you are learning and establishing each new behavior; later on you can require longer time periods to qualify for a larger reward.

Style Change Number 1: Do Not Engage in Any Other Activities While Eating

Many people do other things while they are eating. They watch television, listen to the radio, read the newspaper, or talk on the telephone. These activities reduce the amount of attention paid to the actual act of eating as the attention is shared by two or more events, rather than focused on a single event.

I remember Marsha, an Impulse Eater I worked with several years ago. A young single woman who lived by herself, Marsha loved to talk on the telephone to friends during her meals. The problem was that by entertaining herself in this way she would up taking second, and even third, helpings of food. By not paying attention to the act of eating, she ended up eating more than she intended to and more than she needed to eliminate her hunger.

If you are an Impulse Eater, then, by definition, you are an inattentive eater. This is why it is extremely important for you to no longer do other things while you are eating. You need to develop a new habit of paying attention to eating, something that you will be much more likely to do if you are not distracted with other activities.

Of course, if you live with other people, you probably have conversations with them at the table during meals. While you cannot ignore your family or friends who are sharing mealtimes with you, you must stop any other extraneous activity that is not appropriate at mealtimes if you truly want to turn your weight problem around.

You may argue that if you stop reading that magazine during breakfast or turn off the news at dinner you will be bored during your meals. That's exactly the point. Eating is not a time for entertainment (or at least it shouldn't be), it is a time for nourishment.

Have your entertainment before or after instead of during your meal. You will force yourself to focus more on your eating, thereby decreasing the inattentive, impulsive overeating that has caused you to be overweight.

Style Change Number 2: Always Use Dishes and Utensils When Eating

At first this may sound silly, but if you think about it for a minute you will realize that there are probably many times during the day when you eat without using dishes or utensils.

Many foods can be eaten easily without a spoon, knife, or fork, such as sandwiches, pizza, candy, cookies, snack foods like potato chips, nuts, or pretzels, chicken, burgers, hot dogs, french fries, many types of raw fruits and vegetables, and so on. Many of these foods also do not require a dish—a napkin, or just a hand, suffices.

Because Impulse Eaters do not pay enough attention to the act of eating, it is important for them to take steps to make eating more noteworthy. Complicating the act of eating by using dishes and utensils makes more of an event of a snack or meal.

To take an example from my own past, about twenty-two years ago, when I first started applying the principles outlined in this book to my eating, I remember eating a candy bar, yes, a candy bar, by placing it on a small dish and using a knife and fork. Although this may seem like a strange behavior, let's take a look at what happened as a result of eating the candy bar in this way.

First of all, it certainly made more of an event of eating the candy bar; you are more apt to take note of what you are doing when you put the candy bar on a plate and use utensils than you are when simply eating it straight from the wrapper. By adding complexity to the eating process, it requires more attention.

Second, eating the candy bar in this way is much more time consuming than eating it with your hands. By adding time to the eating process, it has become a more salient, or noteworthy, event. Adding time to the eating process is also helpful in determining when you are full.

Although I do not suggest that you make a habit of eating candy bars even when utilizing this method, there are many other foods that are not, but should be, eaten this way. As a general rule, use a dish and flatware whenever possible.

Style Change Number 3: Eat Slowly

By and large, Impulse Eaters have a bad habit of gobbling their food. They are reaching for their next bite of food before they have even swallowed the one that still is in their mouths. If you are usually the first one done with your meal, there is a good chance that you are gobbling.

For some reason, men seem to be more prone to eating food in this manner than women (this probably has something to do with it being "unladylike" to shovel food into your mouth). I remember working with Matt, an Impulse Eater who ate extremely fast.

To get a better idea of Matt's eating behavior, I brought a tray of food from our cafeteria into the treatment session, so that I could observe him in action. With head bent over plate, and utensils never leaving his hands, Matt consumed the meal in record time.

With my feedback, and a good bit of work, Matt eventually was able to slow down his eating. If you eat quickly, you can do the same.

Just like the other problem behaviors we have discussed in this chapter, how fast you eat is a habit that can be changed. The pace of eating can be slowed down by making a few behavioral changes.

Five ways to slow the pace of eating are:

1. Take small bites. Using a salad fork or teaspoon rather than a dinner fork or tablespoon can, at least initially, help you to take smaller bites.
2. Chew your food slowly.
3. Swallow the food in your mouth before taking another bite.
4. Put down your utensils in between bites.
5. Take short rest breaks during meals.

By slowing the pace of eating you will end up eating less because you will be allowing more time to pass and thereby allow your stomach the time it takes to signal your brain that you are full. Stop eating when you are full or almost full.

This can be a little tricky for Impulse Eaters, since they usually cannot tell when they are full. Therefore, you will have to experiment a bit here. Try to stop eating when you think you have consumed enough food, then wait twenty minutes and see how you feel. You need to wait this period of time because it generally takes about twenty minutes until the brain registers that the stomach is full. If you are still hungry twenty minutes later, you can then eat more. But if you are not, do not eat any more food. (Second portions always must pass the twenty-minute test.)

Try eating progressively less and you will find that you need a lot less food to alleviate hunger than you think. Remember, if you are still hungry after the twenty minutes have passed, you can then eat more. So by waiting, you really are not giving anything up except unnecessary eating.

Another way to eat less is to use a small plate or bowl to make your food portion appear larger than it is. Placing your dinner on a salad or dessert plate rather than a dinner plate tricks the brain by tricking the eye.

USING AVERSIVE IMAGERY

Aversive imagery is actually a form of punishment. As opposed to positive reinforcement, the goal with punishment is to decrease the likelihood or frequency of a behavior by applying something negative to it.

Aversive imagery involves first picturing the undesired behavior in your head and then imagining unpleasant consequences that result from the problem behavior. The negative consequences that are imagined usually are exaggerated or extreme. The idea here is that the more of an impact is made by the imagined consequences, the more likely you will be to develop an aversion to the behavior you want to eliminate.

Aversive techniques, including aversive imagery, have been used for decades to treat many different kinds of impulse-related problems, including sexual and substance-related disorders. The research indicates that these techniques can be helpful in reducing unwanted behaviors if you simultaneously positively reinforce new, desired behaviors.

To use aversive imagery, you must first come up with the images that depict the behaviors you want to decrease. For many Impulse Eaters, this may mean picturing yourself standing up eating food in front of your open refrigerator. Or perhaps you might use the mental image of eating fast food in your car. Maybe eating on the couch while watching television is something you can relate to.

In picking the scenes that you will imagine, use ones that are frequently a problem for you. Trying to get rid of a bad behavior that comes up only once in a while—picking meat off the turkey carcass on Thanksgiving, for instance—is not worthy of your time or attention.

After you have chosen the images that contain the problem behaviors you want to eliminate, you then can begin to think about the aversive consequences that you can incorporate into each scene. For instance, if one of the behaviors you want to reduce is standing in front of the refrigerator eating, you might picture yourself doing this, but then exaggerate it to the point where you see yourself very quickly stuffing food into your face, having food dribbling onto your chin, your stomach bloat up and distend, and then vomiting up the food onto the floor in front of the refrigerator.

While I know this sounds repulsive, it is worth doing because it is effective. By first imaging your problem behavior and then imaging the aversive consequences that it produces, as extreme or as exaggerated as needed to have impact, you will end up suppressing the problem behavior. Pair that with the positive reinforcement you are using to increase your new eating behaviors and you will be well on your way to gaining permanent control over your eating and your weight.

For each image, start with a detailed description of the problem behavior you will imagine and then the aversive consequences resulting from the problem behavior that you will picture in your head.

Problem Behavior

_____

_____

_____

Aversive Consequences for Problem Behavior

_____

_____

_____

Find a quiet, comfortable place where you won't be interrupted. Then follow these directions:

1. Get into a reclining position and close your eyes.
2. Imagine your problem behavior as if it was a movie in your head. To make the scene real, try to invoke all of the sights, sounds, smells, and tastes that would accompany this situation. Imagine the situation for about twenty seconds.
3. Now imagine the aversive consequences that result from your problem behavior, again trying to make it as lifelike as possible. Think of these consequences for about twenty seconds.
4. Stop imagining the scene and relax for about a minute. Then repeat steps 2 and 3.

Although I have listed imagining the problem behavior and the aversive consequences as two different steps, it is important that both of these aspects of the scene converge into one coherent image, or string of related images, rather than two separate unrelated scenes.

By repeatedly imagining the same scene over and over again, the problem behavior will take on the negative emotions associated with the aversive consequences. In other words, you will begin to be repelled by rather than drawn to your problem behavior. Remember, though, the procedure will only work if the aversive consequences you use are truly aversive to you.

You may be tempted to use this technique to try to eliminate your cravings for certain foods. However, unless you also happen to be a Hedonist, your focus needs to be on *how* you eat, not on *what* you eat. Therefore, it is important that you include problem *behaviors* in your scene, not problem *foods*.

There is a scene that one of my patients used on herself that effectively demonstrates the use of this technique.

Hope had a habit of gobbling her food, which was resulting in overeating and weight gain since the faster you eat, the more you eat.

One evening Hope and her husband went out to dinner with another couple whom they did not know very well. The other couple chose the restaurant, one known for serving enormous portions of food. In any event, when the food arrived at the table, everyone proceeded to dig in.

Apparently, Hope was not the only one at the table who had a habit of gobbling. As she watched the eating behavior of her companions, she felt herself repulsed by the way they ate.

Because of the strong negative emotions this experience stirred in her, I suggested that Hope start using it as a mental picture to discourage her own gobbling. She imagined herself eating quickly at the restaurant table and then switched her attention to the behavior of the other couple. As she watched them eat, she grew nauseated and faint.

In this particular scene, not only her behavior, but similar behavior displayed by others, elicited the negative consequences. Although this is a bit different from the standard procedure, the advantage here is that the event actually occurred, making it easy for Hope to conjure up this mental picture.

You also should feel free to incorporate real-life experiences into your scenes, when appropriate. However, don't forget that the most important consideration is that the aversive part of your scene is sufficiently negative, not whether it actually has occurred.

OTHER THINGS YOU SHOULD KNOW ABOUT

Stimulants

Nicotine and caffeine are two common, over-the-counter stimulants. They increase the speed of many of your internal bodily functions and as a consequence make you feel "hyper."

Unfortunately, feeling speeded up lends itself to inattentive and impulsive eating, the very type of eating behavior you are trying so hard to eliminate. Therefore, it's in your best interest to try to reduce or completely avoid the use of stimulants.

I know this is easier said than done. If you are hooked on cigarettes or caffeine you probably will have a very hard time giving either of them up, especially when you are working on your weight. In general, it is usually better to tackle one problem at a time— giving up coffee, quitting smoking, and changing your eating habits are certainly more than anyone should take on all at once.

However, it is important for you to recognize how the use of certain commonly used substances may interfere with achieving your goal. With this knowledge, you can then make your choices from an informed position.

Alcohol

Alcohol can be a serious problem for the Impulse Eater who is trying to get control of his or her eating behavior. Because alcohol serves as a behavioral disinhibitor, it will be substantially more difficult to control your eating behaviors if you are under the influence.

Try to limit your intake of alcohol while you are developing your new eating habits. It is hard enough to make changes in your eating habits without the added disadvantage that this drug produces.

Low Blood Sugar and Gobbling

When you go for a long period of time without eating, your blood-sugar level lowers and you feel an overwhelming urgency to eat. This feeling often leads to uncontrolled, fast eating—the very type of behavior the Impulse Eater is trying to avoid.

Impulse Eaters need to schedule their meals and snacks regularly to avoid extreme lows in blood sugar. Try to space your meals no more than five hours apart, or even more frequently, if necessary. This will keep your blood-sugar level relatively steady so that you avoid a hypoglycemic reaction.

Gaining control over your eating behavior will not be possible if your body is so deprived of food that you are ravenous and out of control. With a little forethought, you can make sure you avoid this problem.

Problem Foods

Although the focus for Impulse Eaters is on eating behaviors, not types of food, there are certain foods that inexplicably seem to trigger fast, uncontrolled eating behavior. Crunchy foods, in particular, fall into this category.

Popcorn is a good example. Most of us are reaching for the next handful of popcorn before we have even swallowed the one in our mouths! That constant hand-to-mouth movement that comes with eating popcorn is the kind of behavior that the Impulse Eater should fight hard to eliminate. Therefore, foods that elicit this kind of eating (popcorn, cereal, chips, etc.) are best avoided, at least until you are well into the maintenance phase of your program.

AFTER COMPLETING THE PROGRAM

Habits are ingrained patterns of behavior that are established over long periods of time. Changing old, unwanted habits into new, more helpful habits also takes some time.

During the treatment program, you will have focused on changing your eating environment and your eating style, and using positive reinforcement and aversive imagery to help strengthen your new habits and weaken your old ones. As a result, you are headed in the right direction.

However, this is only the beginning. The new habits you have started to develop need to become as ingrained as your old patterns of behavior, replacing those inappropriate strategies. In this regard, time will play an important role.

By continuing to use the techniques you have learned in this chapter, you will lose your extra weight. Moreover, because you have eliminated the real cause of your weight problem, you will *stay* thin—not just for a little while, but *forever.*

I still use many of the procedures outlined here today, twenty-two years after my initial weight loss. For example, I still use a small salad-size dish as a dinner plate, and a small fork as a dinner fork. I use aversive imagery to suppress my tendency to gobble. I praise myself for good eating behavior (although I used material rewards extensively when I first lost the weight, praise alone seems to do the trick at this point).

Nobody likes to feel out of control. By being in control of your eating behavior rather than letting it control you, you will gain self-respect, self-confidence, and a new sense of well-being. This is what you deserve, and what you will obtain, not just for now, but for always.

3

The Hedonist:
You Are What You Eat

Mary lives to eat. Of all the pleasures there are in life, eating is her number-one favorite. She particularly loves desserts, and indulges in them daily.

"How will I ever get thin?" Mary asked me when we first met. "I can't give up sweets—I really look forward to them."

"Is there anything else you really enjoy besides desserts?" I asked her.

"Well...I really can't think of anything offhand. Maybe I need a hobby, or to go back to school or work."

Of all the different reasons that people overeat, the reasons of the Hedonist are perhaps the easiest to understand. The Hedonist, quite simply, overeats because of the enjoyment derived from the taste of food.

Obviously, almost all of us obtain some degree of pleasure from the act of eating. Food that tastes good is much more enjoyable to eat than food that does not.

However, enjoying tasty food and developing a *lifestyle* based on eating tasty food are entirely different matters. The Hedonist fits the latter description, food being his or her number-one form of entertainment and pleasure.

There is nothing that the Hedonist likes to do more than eat. Simultaneously, Hedonists are relatively selective about what they eat—they are only interested in food that appeals to their palates. This is not to say that all Hedonists are gourmets; they just have certain categories of food they prefer.

Hedonists tend to concentrate their food selections in two categories—sweets (high-sugar foods) and fats. Some Hedonists overload their diets with high-sugar foods, others with high-fat foods, and some with both types of foods. The problem is that high-sugar and -fat foods usually are very high in calories, which is why Hedonists have such a struggle with their weight.

I remember Patricia, a Hedonist who was addicted to sweets. Patricia "had to have" a dessert following lunch and dinner every day. Although she was twenty pounds overweight and unhappy with her appearance, the idea of giving up even *one* of these desserts was unthinkable to her. She derived immense pleasure from her daily food treats, and was unwilling (at least at first) to give up this small but significant form of daily satisfaction.

When we take a closer look at Patricia's life it becomes easy to see how food came to play such an important role. At forty-five, Patricia has never been married and hasn't had a long-term relationship with a man since college. She lives alone and has only a couple of friends, who really are more acquaintances to share activities with than actual friends. Although she has a number of hobbies and interests, in addition to an interesting career as an attorney, cooking and baking consume much of her free time.

One could hypothesize that the pleasure Patricia derives from food compensates, at least to some extent, for the absence of meaningful relationships in her life. Afraid to trust people, for fear she will get hurt, she is unable to get close enough to other people to establish significant relationships. Unlike relationships, which always carry with them the possibility of experiencing pain, eating is a "safe" alternative way to get pleasure from everyday life.

Until Patricia expanded her world, so that she could receive gratification from close, meaningful relationships with other people, she could not give up her desserts. But once she achieved this goal, her need to get enjoyment from food decreased. Then the weight came off.

If you repeatedly use highly caloric food for pleasure and entertainment, then you probably are a Hedonist. What you are eating is the reason you are overweight.

If you are a Hedonist, you can learn to change your eating pattern. By changing your attitude toward food, and learning how to get enjoyment and pleasure from activities other than eating, you will become the thin person you always have wanted to be.

THE CAUSES OF HEDONISTIC EATING

When I was in graduate school one of my professors presented the results of a study on eating in which rats were the subjects. The animals were given a choice between traditional rat food and chocolate-chip cookies. The results of this taste test were definitive: Nine out of every ten rats preferred the cookies, heading straight for them every time.

What does this tell us? Actually, two different and important things. First of all, the findings from this study suggest that there are taste bud preferences for sweets that are prevalent in other animal species, not just human beings. Second, it indicates that this preference is biological or innate, not learned.

This second point is particularly interesting in that it contradicts the notion that we learn to favor certain types of food through our experiences. The rats, I think we can safely assume, did not have any prior exposure to chocolate-chip cookies, or any type of cookies or sweets, before the experiment began. Because they did not have a history associated with sweets, it is clear that their preference for this type of food was automatic and innate.

Many years later a similar experiment was conducted with high-fat foods. Similar results were obtained—when given the choice, rats prefer high-fat food to rat food.

The findings from these two studies pose potential problems for overweight people who consume a lot of sweets or fats. If we, by our very nature as human animals, have an innate preference for high-calorie foods, how are we going to successfully reduce our intake of them? In other words, how can we overcome our true nature?

Luckily, there are several highly effective ways to deal with our tendency to prefer these foods, and these methods form the foundation of the treatment program for the Hedonist. However, before we get to these, I'd like to discuss one other important factor that contributes to overindulging in high-sugar and high-fat foods.

By definition, Hedonists follow a pleasure-seeking approach to life, rather than one of self-discipline and self-denial. This style of living is *learned,* and therefore can be unlearned.

Essentially, the hedonistic approach to eating is undisciplined. Hedonists follow the motto, "If it feels good, do it," and when applied to their food this translates into "If it tastes good, eat it." But this lack of self-control has negative consequences—not only do Hedonists weigh more than they want to, they may secretly have bad feelings about themselves because of their undisciplined behavior (although, on the other hand, some Hedonists are very good at rationalizing their indulgences).

Although we do not have the power to alter our innate chemistry (we may always prefer chocolate-chip cookies to carrots), we do have the ability to monitor and restrict our own behavior, despite our desires and preferences. The fact that many adults maintain monogamous sexual relationships in the face of temptation attests to our ability to control our biological urges.

In summary, the Hedonist is a product of nature *and* nurture. As with most human problems, there are both biological (innate) and environmental (learned) components to this pattern of behavior. While current technology does not yet allow us to alter our inherent taste preferences, we can alter the manner in which we live, and, in this way, control our weight and our lives.

THE PSYCHOLOGICAL APPROACH TO HEDONISTIC EATING

The Program for the Hedonist includes four specific treatment techniques that will eliminate this type of overeating. Two of the procedures directly address the overconsumption of highly caloric foods, while the other two techniques focus on thoughts and behaviors that will promote a new healthier lifestyle.

To reduce your intake of highly caloric foods, you will learn how to use food substitution to replace high-calorie foods with lower-calorie alternatives, and portion control to decrease the amount of food you consume.

Program for the Hedonist

Treatment Method	Begin
Food substitution	Week 1
Portion control	Week 2
Gaining pleasure from alternative activities	Week 3
Developing a healthy food attitude	Week 4

To be successful at weight control, Hedonists must also deal with broader lifestyle issues, developing the ability to gain pleasure from activities other than eating and taking on new, healthier attitudes toward food (learning to put food in its proper perspective).

Before beginning the treatment program, you need to collect detailed information about your eating habits. This information will be very useful as you learn each of the treatment techniques.

Complete the Daily Food Log on page 35 in chapter 2 for at least a week, keeping a detailed record of all of the sweets and high-fat foods you eat. You don't have to list everything you eat (unless you also happen to be an Impulse Eater), just food that falls into the high-sugar or high-fat category.

If you have trouble distinguishing what is and what is not a high-sugar food, the following list contains items that are high in sugar:

Cookies	Doughnuts
Cake	Soda
Pies, tarts, and cobblers	Ice cream
Candy	Milk shakes
Gelatin desserts	Sherbet, sorbet, and ices
Pudding and custard	Granola bars
Sweet muffins (e.g., blueberry)	Toaster tarts
	Sweetened cereal
Chocolate	Jelly and jam

Remember, what we are concerned about here are *calories*, not sugar per se. Therefore, you should check out the calorie content of your favorite sweets, either by looking at the nutritional facts panel on the food's package, or by consulting a calorie book.

If your problem foods tend to be those high in fat, you can get detailed information on the fat content of a particular food by looking at the number of fat grams, or the percentage of calories obtained from fat, it contains. This information is also included on the nutritional facts panel for most foods, or you can get it from a nutritional guidebook (some books contain calories as well as a detailed nutritional breakdown, giving you all the information that you will ever need).

Following is a list of foods that are very high in fat:

Nuts, including peanut butter
Butter, margarine, and oil
    (all types)
Fried foods
Heavy cream
Whipped cream
Sour cream
Mayonnaise
Salad dressings (except
    low/no fat)
Bacon
Sausage

Most cheeses (except feta,
    ricotta, and low fat)
Frankfurters
Potato chips, corn chips,
    tortilla chips
Ham
Bologna
Salami
Pastrami
Duck
Pâté
Ribs

Of course, there are a number of foods that are high in both fat and sugar (e.g., ice cream) that could easily appear on both of our "problem food lists." Now that you have a pretty good idea which foods are your problem foods, let's turn to the tools you will use to change what you eat.

TRICKING YOUR TASTE BUDS WITH FOOD SUBSTITUTION

If you love sweet foods you are always going to love sweet foods, so you are doomed to stay overweight, right? Wrong. It is not the food that you love but the *taste* of that food, in this case, the taste of "sweet." That is where at least part of the answer comes in: You can satisfy your need to experience a sweet taste without consuming highly caloric foods by using the method of *food substitution*.

Quite simply, food substitution is the process of replacing problem foods with lower-calorie alternatives that provide a similar taste sensation. The alternatives can be reduced-fat or reduced-sugar foods (e.g., reduced-fat milk), foods that contain fat or sugar substitutes (e.g., Olean, NutraSweet), or entirely different foods that have similar taste appeal, but are naturally lower in calories (e.g., an orange for orange sherbert).

The most obvious examples of food substitution come from the large assortment of low-fat, reduced-fat, and fat-free products readily available in supermarkets today. There is reduced-fat mayonnaise, low-fat sour cream, reduced-fat hot dogs, fat-free popcorn, etc., all designed to provide similar taste experiences with lower fat content and fewer calories.

In addition, just recently, the first fat substitute (Olean) has entered the market. While at the time of writing this chapter, the fat substitute is available only in chips, I expect it will be much more prevalent, included as an ingredient in a variety of food products, by the time you read this.

Likewise, reduced-sugar foods (i.e., "half the sugar") and products containing sugar substitutes, such as NutraSweet, can successfully fill in for high-calorie, sugar-laden foods. Many of these foods taste very good, perhaps almost as good as their more fattening counterparts.

Eating reduced-fat and reduced-sugar foods, as well as foods containing fat and sugar substitutes, will automatically decrease the amount of calories you take in.

For some Hedonists, though, there is a tendency to consume *more* of a product when it contains reduced fat or sugar, or fat/sugar substitutes. For instance, the usual tablespoon of sour cream on top of the baked potato is replaced by reduced-fat sour cream, but now a *heaping* tablespoon (equivalent to *two* tablespoons) is used. Or the handful of regular potato chips you used to enjoy on occasion turns into a bag a day of the new fat-free chips. In these situations just as many or more calories end up being consumed by using lower-calorie foods.

This may occur for one of two reasons. The first reason is that many people fool themselves into thinking they can have more of a lower-calorie product because it has fewer calories. This, of course, is not true; eat enough of a low-calorie food and it becomes "high calorie."

Sara is a good example of someone who did this. She was a Hedonist who could not replace foods with lower-calorie substitutes—she would simply increase her intake so that she ended up eating just as many or more calories. She would purchase a reduced-calorie bakery-style cake at her supermarket. Because the cake was low calorie—only 120 calories per slice—somehow she figured that meant she could have several slices a day.

The second reason that I think people tend to eat more of some reduced-fat and reduced-sugar foods (the sugar and fat substitute products are less likely to fall into this category) is because they need greater amounts of these foods to get the taste sensation they are after. I recently purchased a reduced-calorie strawberry jam to substitute for my regular higher-calorie strawberry jam at breakfast. Although I knew better, I found that I was using *more than three times* as much of the new product because it was much less sweet than my usual jam. I subsequently went back to my old favorite, where I actually was taking in fewer calories.

Not all Hedonists respond like Sara or myself. However, I have seen it happen frequently enough that I feel I should alert you to this possibility.

An alternative to replacing high-fat, high-sugar foods with reduced-fat, reduced-sugar foods, or fat or sugar substitutes, is to replace high-calorie foods with entirely different foods that are lower in calories, but serve similar taste functions. Let me give you a few examples here.

I have to admit that I love high-fat foods—particularly anything with cheese or sauces on it (pizza, fettucini Alfredo, nachos), and everything fried (french fries, fried chicken). However, since I also love being a size 6, I learned how to trick my taste buds into being satisfied with naturally lower-calorie alternatives.

Case in point: my ricotta pizza. I have always loved pizza, but the mozzarella cheese and oil-laden tomato sauce covering the pie were definite no-nos. Fortunately for me many Italian restaurants and pizza shops now offer individual gourmet pizzas for one, where you can select exactly what you want on your pie. When I order mine I ask for ricotta cheese and vegetables only—no sauce, no mozzarella cheese, no Parmesan cheese—just ricotta cheese and vegetables on pizza crust.

Since the vegetables are usually sautéed in olive oil and garlic, I can't say this is an entirely fat-free creation. But then that's really not the point. The point is to decrease the *number of calories* consumed, and my pizza alternative is less than one-half the calories of a regular pie. It satisfies my craving for pizza without sacrificing my figure.

Remember Patricia, the sweet-loving Hedonist I introduced you to at the beginning of this chapter? The one who had to have a dessert after every lunch and every dinner?

I acquainted Patricia with the same trick I have been using on myself for years (yes, I love desserts almost as much as I love high-fat foods). The secret is this: one peppermint hard candy after every meal. That's right, that red-and-white hard candy serves as my after-lunch and after-dinner dessert, giving me the intensely sweet taste of sugar that I crave after a meal without adding more than a few calories (each is about twenty-five calories).

At this point I can hear you saying, "One peppermint does not a dessert make," and you would be right. But remember, it is not the food itself that the Hedonist is stuck on, but the taste it creates. The peppermint is not intended to fill you up (the food you ate during your meal should have done that), but to meet a specific taste need that, for whatever reason, some people seem to require.

Another food I often use as a substitute for a sweet is an orange. For me, a ripe orange has an intensely sweet taste that I find very satisfying.

You can switch to reduced-fat and reduced-sugar foods and the fat and sugar substitutes I talked about earlier, and if that works for you, great. But if you are like a lot of other Hedonists, and these replacements just end up in your eating more and consuming the same amount of calories, then you should consider using the alternative food approach, replacing high-calorie foods with entirely different foods that have a similar effect on your palate.

The list below includes a few examples of foods (some reduced fat and sugar, some containing fat and sugar replacements, and some naturally low-calorie alternatives) that I have found work well as replacements for high-calorie foods. Try those that you think might do the trick for you—but feel free to get creative and come up with some ideas of your own.

Sample Food Substitutes and Alternatives

For	Substitute
Chocolate	Chocolate-flavored hard candy *or* diet hot cocoa *or* diet chocolate Popsicle
Ice cream	Frozen yogurt *or* fruit ice Popsicle *or* low-calorie milk shake
Potato chips	Nonfat popcorn *or* rice cakes
Sour cream	Low-fat cottage cheese
Salad dressing	Balsamic vinegar *or* yogurt-based dressing

Now look at the Daily Food Log form you filled out earlier. Note your problem foods, and try to come up with alternative foods you can use as lower calorie replacements.

As a Hedonist, you are overweight because you make bad food choices. Of the five different eating profiles, yours demands you make changes in *what* you eat. Whether you use reduced-fat and -sugar products, foods containing fat or sugar substitutes, or foods that are naturally lower in calories (or some combination of the three), you must begin immediately to replace high-calorie foods with lower-calorie alternatives.

HAVING YOUR CAKE AND EATING IT TOO

Another way to deal with the taste bud problem is to give yourself some of the high-calorie foods you desire but strictly limit the size of your portions. This way you actually can "have your cake and eat it too." It's just that you now only get a sliver of cake, not a gigantic slice.

By decreasing the size of your potions you will significantly decrease the number of calories you consume. But how can you be content with less, when you really want more?

The answer is to make less seem like more. By eating the problem food very, very slowly, and savoring each and every morsel, you can trick yourself into being satisfied with smaller portions.

The technique works for two reasons. First, by eating slowly you increase the amount of time it takes you to eat. The total time you spend eating the food ends up being about the same as it would had you eaten your usual amount of food in your usual way. By taking the same amount of time to eat, you trick your body into thinking you have had enough.

Second, by making a big deal out of each bite—chewing the food slowly, rolling it around in your mouth—you get more "bang for your buck" (or bang for your bite, in this case). The amount of taste you get is increased because the food is in your mouth longer. Your taste quota is met with less food.

No, your stomach won't be as full as it would with larger portions, but you can easily fill up on other nonproblematic foods if you need to. This should not be a problem, though. Remember, for the Hedonist the issue is taste, not hunger. The taste of the food and the resulting pleasure that it produces are what lead the Hedonist to eat, not the sensation of hunger or feeling of fullness experienced in the stomach.

One of the foods that I love most in the world is Fig Newton cookies. From time to time, I allow myself one cookie. I eat it extremely slowly and relish every bite. By eating it this way it probably is like someone else eating three cookies. The time it takes for me to eat my one cookie, plus the amount of taste satisfaction I get because of the way I eat it (savoring each crumb), enables me to be satisfied with just one.

Make a game out of it—see *how long* it can take you to eat that smaller portion. You will see that less can actually be more!

ARE WE HAVING FUN YET?

If you were to take a poll of one hundred Hedonists, chances are that at least ninety would admit that eating is their most enjoyable activity. Most Hedonists depend on food to bring pleasure to each and every day.

As we have discussed, Hedonists must make changes in what they eat to achieve lifelong weight control. However, while these changes are necessary conditions for weight control, they are not sufficient in and of themselves. To get thin and stay thin Hedonists also must learn how to get pleasure from activities other than eating.

Granted, we have already acknowledged that you probably place eating as number one on your list of enjoyable activities. But what about those things that you would put in the number-two, -three, and -four spots? What else do you like to do, or what would you like to try doing?

You may already know what types of activities bring you pleasure. If you do, then you are one step ahead of the game. But what if you really haven't thought about your life in this way? What if you really don't know, or haven't explored, what you like to do?

Because of the time that college, graduate school, postgraduate work, and then my career, took out of my life, there were many things that I used to like to do that I seemed to forget about as I grew older. There was a time when I balanced my academic interests with creative and artistic activities, spending my time playing the piano, studying ballet, drawing, baking, and sewing.

In my thirties, when I was comfortably established in my career, I asked myself what happened to that part of me. The answer was that that artistic and creative girl had not vanished. She just went undercover for a while.

Interestingly, when I began to get back into some of these activities in adulthood, I found they had positive effects on many aspects of my life. I seemed to have a broader perspective on my work, more energy, less interest in food, and more enthusiasm for my free time. Why not? Now I had something other than food and work to look forward to.

Do you remember things that you used to enjoy doing? Are there hobbies, interests, or goals you have pushed aside because you have gotten too involved with other things? Putting eating aside, how would you plan out a perfect day—what would you be doing?

As a Hedonist you demand, and need, pleasure in your daily life. To conquer your weight problem once and for all, you will need to make a conscious, concerted effort to incorporate pleasurable activities and events into each and every day.

At first, substituting alternative pleasurable activities for eating will seem like a very sorry substitute. That is because you are in the habit of looking toward food as your pleasure giver. After you have spent some time developing your new approach, you will find that you look toward other types of activities to bring you pleasure and joy. Eventually, you will no longer miss your old way of doing things because now you will have a new, better way—one that gives you pleasure and doesn't put on weight!

Twenty-two years ago I followed the same advice that I am giving you. I made a list of alternative pleasurable activities to substitute for pleasure eating. Instead of dessert after dinner, I took a walk. Instead of a candy bar in the middle of the afternoon, I had a cup of hot tea and read a chapter from a mystery novel. In other words, I used other pleasures in place of my sweets.

Giving up smoking several years ago brought up many of the old battles that I originally had fought when I tackled my weight problem. Giving up cigarettes was similar to what I went through when I reduced my intake of sweets, but even more difficult. I indulged in smoking much more frequently than I did sweets—I had a cigarette on the average of once every twenty to thirty minutes while I was awake. For many years, there was nothing that I had enjoyed as much as smoking (and, I am ashamed to admit, I intentionally increased my smoking as a pleasure substitute when I cut down on the eating), and now I was going to have to find something to give myself some joy on a very frequent basis.

Of course, I could have gone back to sweets. Actually, for a few months, I did just that. But as I saw myself getting larger, I remembered how I used to feel about myself in my overweight days. I would not accept a nonsmoking fat self in place of my previously thin smoking self. Nor would I go back to smoking. I would attack my love of nicotine the same way I conquered my love of sweets.

There was one small, additional problem, though. Many of the things that I enjoyed doing I strongly associated with smoking. When I gardened, I smoked. When I sewed, I smoked. When I read, I smoked.

Because of these associations, I decided to pursue new activities, some that I always thought I might enjoy and others that I just took up on the chance I might like them. And guess what! Lo and behold, no more cigarettes and no more sweets—I was now getting enjoyment from other, new activities.

It took some time and it wasn't easy, but the payoff has been tremendous. Because I have expanded my interests, I have expanded my life—new passions, new friends to share these passions with, new enthusiasm for life. Moreover, I don't need a sugar or nicotine "high" to feel good—I feel good because of what *I do,* not because of food or drugs.

Before you can begin to substitute noneating events for food, you need to be armed with the activities you will use as alternatives. Use the form on page 66 to list pleasurable activities that you will use as alternatives to eating. You can use activities that you currently enjoy, those that you used to enjoy and might like to pursue again, and others that you might want to try for the first time.

Pleasurable Activities

1. _____

2. _____

3. _____

4. _____

5. _____

6. _____

7. _____

8. _____

9. _____

10. _____

Go back to your Daily Food Log to see what times you typically eat your problem foods—those are the times you are going to have to reach for an alternative. Substitute one of your pleasurable alternative activities at the time that you normally would be indulging in your high-calorie food.

Obviously, if your problem food usually comes up during a meal, you are not going to get up and leave your family sitting at the kitchen table while you go take a bubble bath, or do some other type of alternative pleasurable activity. As soon as possible after the meal, you need to give yourself some alternative form of pleasure.

I will never forget Gary, a Hedonist who decided he would substitute sex with his wife for his after-dinner ice cream. Not only did Gary lose weight, he improved his relationship with his wife!

It really doesn't matter which activities you use as long as they make you feel good. Remember, the Hedonist is overweight because he or she uses food to generate pleasure. By learning to rely on non-eating activities to fill this need, you will reduce your intake of problem foods and lose weight.

HOW TO PUT FOOD IN ITS PROPER PERSPECTIVE

Do you eat to live, or live to eat? If you are a Hedonist, you already know the answer to this question—you live to eat. And like most

Hedonists, you probably can't imagine living any other way. But like most things, your attitude toward food is a belief that you have acquired over time.

There are many experiences that contribute to how we view food, but perhaps none influence us as much as our parents' attitudes and behavior toward eating. Parents (usually mothers) set the stage for our understanding of the purpose and place of eating in our lives.

As children, it is our parents who determine when and what we eat. Many families have set mealtimes and discourage snacking between meals. They teach their children that food supplies important nutrients that nourish and energize the body and stress the importance of eating on a regular basis. These types of families usually also are nutrition oriented, providing their children with healthy foods and a well-balanced diet.

Other types of families, for a variety of reasons, do not follow a strict routine for mealtimes. Children are often left to their own devices—eating what they want, whenever they want it. This type of haphazard attitude toward eating is a potential breeding ground for the Hedonist.

In addition, parents, through their own behavior, serve as important examples and role models for their children. Did your parents use food as a form of entertainment? Was eating something they relied on to give them happiness and pleasure? Did they frequently give in to their urges for fattening foods?

Although, in the past, you may have learned to view food's primary function as providing pleasure and entertainment, you now can develop a healthier attitude toward eating.

Changing your attitude toward food works hand in hand with the treatment techniques we have already covered. It will be much easier for you to use the food substitution method, reduce your portions of problematic foods, and replace eating with alternative pleasurable activities, if you believe that the purpose of food is to provide nutrients and energy for the body, not to make you feel good. (You should also note that this can work in the reverse—changing your behavior through using the three procedures can, consequently, produce an attitude change.)

How do you change your attitude toward food? Well, since an attitude really consists of thoughts in our head (comprising how we think of something), the most direct way to alter an attitude is to tackle these thoughts. By modifying the kinds of things that we say to ourselves we can develop new, healthier ways of looking at food.

To change your attitude about food you first need to identify the unhelpful thoughts you have, so that you then can replace them with more helpful thoughts. Moreover, you will need to be able to identify your unhelpful thoughts about food as they are occurring. This will take a bit of practice.

The unhelpful thoughts that Hedonists have about food usually involve enjoyment, pleasure, and entertainment—for example, "a hot fudge sundae will really taste good," "it will be really fun to go out for Italian food," "I could really go for a chocolate bar right now." By first attending to them as they are happening, and then replacing them with new thoughts that reflect a healthier attitude toward food, you will be able to change the way you currently think about food.

To identify your unhelpful thoughts about food, make photocopies of the Daily Food Thoughts form below and complete a new sheet each day. If you find that you are having a hard time identifying your thoughts, try paying attention to your food urges. Food urges usually are triggered by unhelpful thoughts; if you attend to your urges you often can then "backtrack" to your thoughts.

Daily Food Thoughts

Date:_____

Thoughts About Food:

_____

_____

_____

_____

_____

_____

_____

_____

_____

The next step in the process of changing your food attitude is to substitute helpful thoughts for the unhelpful ones you just identified. You will change your thoughts by noticing the problematic ones as they are happening, and immediately replace them with the new, helpful thoughts.

For instance, if you think, "Dessert would really finish off this meal perfectly," you might counter that thought with: "Dessert is full of sugar and calories and has little nutritional value," or "I had enough to eat from my meal, I don't need dessert."

Although initially you may find that you are arguing with yourself quite often, not really believing the new thoughts, eventually you will adopt them as your own. Eventually the new healthier thoughts will pop up automatically, without intentionally conjuring them up or talking yourself into them. If you think of your new thoughts as a new habit, just like any other habit, it is easy to understand how practice eventually produces these results.

I remember when I worked with Deirdre, a Hedonist with a love of chocolate. When she did her daily thought monitoring, it soon became clear that she was having very frequent thoughts and urges for chocolate, which she generally gave in to. In order to work on changing her attitude about this particular food, we developed the following defense for her chocolate attacks: "The only point of chocolate is to make me feel good. I don't use food anymore to make me feel good. I feel good by doing things that interest me and spending time with the important people in my life."

It took some time, but after a few months of practice, Deirdre lost a good deal of her desire for chocolate. In a sense, she had "talked herself out of it" by changing the kinds of things she said in her head. She had changed her attitude about chocolate.

Beth, a Hedonist with a yen for high-fat snack foods, used a slightly different approach. In countering her problem thoughts about chips, peanuts, and other munchies, she embellished and exaggerated the negative aspects of these foods: "Those chips are dripping in oil. They are disgusting, and they will clog up my arteries."

Basically, Beth "grossed herself out" in order to oppose her desire for chips. After repeatedly using this approach, she very rarely has urges for these kinds of foods. Her attitude has changed for the better.

Using some of the thoughts you recorded on your Daily Food Thoughts forms, come up with alternative, helpful thoughts that you can use to counter your problematic thoughts about food.

Problem Thought:

_____

_____

_____

Counterthought:

_____

_____

_____

By changing the types of things you say to yourself, you will change your attitude about food. And by changing your attitude about food, you will find it much easier to resist the high-calorie foods that you have been using inappropriately for pleasure and entertainment.

OTHER THINGS YOU SHOULD KNOW ABOUT

Stimulants

Hedonists who use caffeine or nicotine may find they increase their use of these substances as they decrease their intake of high-calorie foods. Since these substances are used to make you feel good, it is easy to use them to get the lift you now miss from giving up your high-fat and high-sugar foods.

The main problem with doing this (besides the obvious health risks) is that psychoactive substances like these will stand in the way of your learning new skills. Why should you learn how to get pleasure from alternative activities if you can simply drink more coffee or smoke more cigarettes and feel good?

Be careful that you don't fall into this potential pitfall. Learn and rely on the treatment methods in this chapter rather than turning to stimulants.

Alcohol

Like stimulants, alcohol can become an easy substitute for the pleasure-seeking Hedonist. If you enjoy alcoholic beverages, be careful that you don't increase your alcohol consumption as you decrease your eating. Remember, the idea here is to learn how to get pleasure and enjoyment from other activities, not to exchange one bad habit for another.

Low Blood Sugar

It is highly advisable that you eat on a regular basis to avoid extreme lows in your blood-sugar level. When you go for too long a period of time without eating, you may end up experiencing an overwhelming urge to eat. When Hedonists feel this way, they typically reach for their favorite high-calorie foods.

To avoid this potential problem, try to schedule your meals on a regular basis, with four to five hours in between meals. The likelihood of your following this program, and remaining in control, will be much better if you keep a relatively steady blood-sugar level.

Hormones and Food Urges

For female Hedonists, the week or so before the menstrual period is a particularly difficult time. Many women, even those without eating problems, experience an increased desire for highly caloric foods (usually sweets) for a few days prior to the onset of their periods.

These urges, by and large, are caused by hormonal changes. However, knowing that there is a biological basis to this doesn't make it any easier for the Hedonist, who generally has a difficult time saying no to high-calorie foods. For this reason, premenstrual Hedonists have to be particularly on guard using the variety of treatment methods outlined in this chapter.

AFTER COMPLETING THE PROGRAM

The desire to experience pleasure is human nature. For the Hedonist, however, experiencing pleasure translates into eating highly caloric foods.

As you have learned in this program, to get thin and stay thin Hedonists must not only change what they eat by making food substitutions and decreasing the size of their portions, they need to adjust their attitudes and change their behavior so that food plays a less prominent role in their lives.

Hedonism is not a condition that goes away. It's an individual trait that needs to be managed by exercising discipline and control over the way that you live your life. The techniques you have mastered will help you do this not only for your weight but also, if you choose, with other excesses or problem behaviors you want to eliminate.

In conquering my own weight problem, I had to confront my hedonistic tendencies. I often used food for pleasure and entertainment, frequently indulging in high-fat and high-sugar foods. I can honestly say that I no longer turn to eating as my primary source of pleasure. In fact, it is seldom that I eat highly caloric foods, and if I do eat them I use portion control. I now look at food as fuel for my body, and view activities and relationships, not eating, as my sources of pleasure and entertainment.

Obviously, I have had many years to adjust my attitude and behavior. But with practice and persistence you too will achieve your goal.

Just like me, you will not only lose the extra weight, but you will keep it off. This time around you really will be successful, because you will have finally gotten to the heart of your problem.

4

The Stress Reducer:
Stress Busting Is Fat Busting

Jenny is desperate. She's been putting on weight ever since she gave up smoking. She used to use cigarettes to relax but now overeats instead. She thought her eating eventually would normalize as time went on, but it's been three years now and the number on the scale still is going up.

"What am I going to do about my weight?" she asked me at our first session. "Every time I'm stressed out, I end up eating."

"Apparently you have trouble dealing with stress and anxiety. You haven't solved your real problem—your anxiety—you're just using a different substance to try to eliminate it," I replied.

Jenny, like millions of overweight people, uses food as a way to deal with stress. In her case eating, and her weight, became a problem after she quit smoking. Rather than learning how to cope with and minimize the effects of tension, Jenny has replaced one bad habit with another. Until she tackles her stress problem head-on, she'll keep putting on weight.

As you saw in chapter 1, Stress Reducers use food to decrease tension and to relax. When their anxiety increases, so does their eating. Anxiety serves as an emotional trigger for eating.

Many people use food occasionally to try to calm down or relax when they are tense. It can be a way of soothing ourselves during difficult or stressful times. However, some people do this on a regular basis, frequently turning to food to unwind from the stresses and strains of daily life. These are the people who are Stress Reducers.

Our everyday lives generally are filled with minor (and sometimes major) upsets and stresses. Driving to work on the highway, taking care of children, having conflicts with family or friends, having things go wrong with our homes—all of these can be sources of anxiety and discomfort.

For the Stress Reducer, feeling tense is a summons to the refrigerator. Many times, the Stress Reducer is not even aware of what he or she is doing. The behavior is so automatic that it is virtually ignored.

The psychological approach to overeating for the Stress Reducer does not deal with food choices. That's because what you are eating is not the cause of your weight problem, unless you also happen to be a Hedonist. *Why* you are eating—in response to anxiety—is the reason you are overweight.

By learning how to deal with anxiety straight on, rather than trying to suppress it with food, Stress Reducers eliminate the underlying cause of their weight problem.

But before we get to the treatment program, let's talk about some of the predominant causes of anxiety problems and anxious overeating.

THE CAUSES OF ANXIOUS OVEREATING

Because of genetic factors, personality variables, and life experiences, certain people are more likely than others to experience anxiety and tension, and, therefore, are more at risk for becoming Stress Reducers.

To a great extent, the tendency to be anxious is determined by birth. Many people are born with a predisposition to having these feelings.

Studies of identical and fraternal twins raised in different families have looked at the role of genetics in anxiety. This research has shown that identical twins (who are genetically exactly the same) are much more likely than fraternal twins (who are no more genetically alike than nontwin siblings) to have similar levels of anxiety. This clearly indicates that there is a genetic component to anxiety.

Recent research looking at the temperaments of infants suggests early signs exist that can point to an anxious personality. Babies who have trouble adapting to new situations are particularly at risk for having anxiety problems as children and adolescents.

In addition to genes and temperament, our environment can add to the probability of developing a tendency toward anxiety. Through observation of our parents during childhood, we can learn to relate to the world fearfully. For example, if your mother is afraid of heights, you may learn to be afraid of heights. If your father is always warning you about bad things that might happen, you may also develop an apprehensive way of looking at the world.

The fact that anxiety runs in families was clearly demonstrated in a study I conducted in the eighties. Mental-health histories on the relatives of anxious children, hyperactive children, and normal children were collected. As expected, results showed that anxiety problems were much more prevalent in the families of the anxious children than in those of the other two groups of youngsters. In other words, people who have anxious relatives are very likely to be anxious themselves.

As you can see, the tendency to be tense or high strung clearly is not the "fault" of those people affected; genetic and environmental components largely determine who will and who will not be anxious. However, although anxious people are not responsible for the presence of this trait, it does become their job to moderate its effect. In my clinical practice, I refer to this as "playing the hand you are dealt."

You can manage your anxiety by using substance-oriented methods, such as food, for reducing your tension, or you can learn more adaptive coping strategies and be thin. The psychological treatment of anxiety-related overeating supports this second approach, showing you how to permanently control your weight by eliminating the true source of your weight problem.

Let's turn to it now.

THE PSYCHOLOGICAL APPROACH
TO ANXIOUS OVEREATING

If anxiety is playing a role in your eating, you must stop using food in this way if you want to gain permanent control over your weight. The way to do this is to get rid of the anxiety. By developing psychological skills that reduce tension and increase relaxation, anxiety-triggered overeating disappears because the cue or signal that elicits eating has vanished.

The Program for the Stress Reducer lists the psychological self-help techniques you can use to decrease anxiety and increase relaxation. The procedures include two that focus on feelings, two that focus on thoughts, and one that deals with behavior.

In order to reduce the uncomfortable physical feelings of anxiety, you will learn deep muscle relaxation and abdominal breathing. To eliminate anxious styles of thinking, you will use coping self-statements and thought-stopping techniques. Last, you will overcome your fearful behavior with exposure.

Program for the Stress Reducer

Treatment Method	Begin
Deep muscle relaxation	Week 1
Abdominal breathing	Week 2
Coping self-statements	Week 3
Thought-stopping	Week 4
Exposure	Week 5

The chart also includes a schedule for learning the techniques. It is best to follow the specific order indicated for developing the skills: Most people find it's easiest to learn them in this sequence, and some of the procedures rely on your having acquired the other (earlier) skills.

The techniques should be tackled one by one, allowing ample time to become comfortable using a procedure before moving on to the next one. As you can see, I recommend that you set aside five weeks to learn all of the anxiety-reduction methods. Although this may seem like a long time (I know you're eager to see the weight come off!), experience has shown that to really become good at using the techniques, and to maintain them as lifelong skills, you need to make the initial time investment. Isn't it worth a few weeks of your life to change the way you look and feel forever?

By using your new skills you will eliminate the cause of your overeating and excess weight. As you stop using food in response to tension and anxiety, you will lose weight and become thin. Moreover, you will *stay* thin because you will have permanently erased the source of your weight problem: anxiety-triggered overeating.

ELIMINATING FEELINGS OF TENSION

There are many different kinds of anxious feelings. Some people feel generally jittery or tense, while others experience tension as localized physical problems like headaches, neck stiffness, or stomachaches. In extreme cases, bodily tension can be experienced to such a large degree that the person ends up having panic attacks.

Whether you have generalized or localized physical signs of anxiety, you will experience major benefits from using relaxation techniques. Relaxation produces physiological changes that counter those you feel while under stress. These include decreasing your heart, metabolic, and breathing (respiration) rates, reducing your blood pressure, and alleviating muscle tension.

In addition to these measurable changes, relaxation has many other pluses:

- Decreasing your overall level of arousal
- Increasing your tolerance for stressful events
- Improving your attention and concentration
- Reducing fatigue
- Improving your sleep
- Reducing stress-related aches and pains
- Decreasing anxiety-triggered overeating

There are two procedures that are particularly helpful for countering the uncomfortable effects that stress and tension have on the body. The first method is deep muscle relaxation, and the second is abdominal breathing. Let's begin with deep muscle relaxation.

Deep Muscle Relaxation

Deep muscle relaxation involves tightening and then relaxing the various muscles in your body. One by one, each muscle first is tensed for a specified period of time, and then relaxed. In this way the procedure teaches you to identify whether your muscles are tense or relaxed, and how to move from the one state, muscular tension, to the other, muscular relaxation.

This technique first attracted attention when mental-health professionals began using it in the 1950s. At that time, the procedure was used in conjunction with other psychological treatments to successfully eliminate fears and phobias. Since then researchers have discovered that deep muscle relaxation is a beneficial procedure by itself for reducing generalized or "free-floating" anxiety—the type of anxiety commonly experienced by anxiety-triggered overeaters.

In order to become proficient in this technique, you must begin by practicing it once a day. The exercises do not take long to do, and, believe me, they are well worth the effort.

It's best to schedule your practice sessions when you will not be disturbed by other activities in your household (for example, when you first wake up in the morning or before you go to sleep at night). Set aside about twenty minutes to do them.

Wear loose, comfortable clothing and get into a reclining position—lying on top of your bed, stretched out on the sofa, or in a reclining armchair. If you wear glasses, it's best to remove them before doing the exercises.

1. Close your eyes. Now take three deep, slow breaths. To yourself (not out loud) say, "calm," "relax," or "let go" (pick one—this will be your *key word*) as you exhale.
2. Stretch your arms straight out from your body and clench both of your fists very tightly. Feel the uncomfortable feelings in your forearms, triceps, and hands. Hold the tension for about ten seconds, and then all of a sudden "let go" (use your *key word*), releasing all the tension and just letting your arms flop down to your sides. Notice the difference between the relaxed state of these muscles and the tension you experienced a few seconds ago. Continue to relax for about fifteen seconds. Now repeat the exercise one more time.

(*Note:* All of the exercises use the same time periods for tensing and relaxing muscles—ten seconds for tension and fifteen seconds for relaxation.)

3. Bend your arms at the elbows, bringing your hands up to your shoulders. Your fingers need to be extended straight up, toward your head. Feel the tension in your biceps and hands. Hold this position, and then relax (*key word*). Repeat.

4. Shrug your shoulders up toward your ears. Hold this position, concentrating on the tension you experience, and then relax (*key word*). Repeat.

5. Arch your shoulders back, lifting your upper back off the surface you are lying on. Feel the tension, and then let go (*key word*). Repeat.

6. Extend your legs straight out, pointing your toes. Notice the tightness in your thighs, calves, and feet. Hold this position and then relax (*key word*). Repeat.

7. Extend your legs straight out, flexing your toes (pointing them toward your head). Feel the tension in your legs, and then relax (*key word*). Repeat.

8. Push your chin into your chest, feeling the tightness in your neck and upper back muscles. Hold and then let go (*key word*). Repeat.

9. Push your head back, as if you were trying to touch the back of your head to your upper back. Hold and then relax (*key word*). Repeat.

10. Raise your eyebrows up as high as they will go. Feel the tension in your forehead. Hold this position, and then relax (*key word*). Repeat.

11. Clench your lips and teeth together tightly. Feel the tension in your jaw and the muscles around your mouth. Concentrate on the unpleasant feelings, and then let go (*key word*). Repeat.

12. Open your mouth as wide as you can. Hold the tension, and then relax (*key word*). Repeat.

13. Carefully squeeze your eyelids shut. Feel the uncomfortable sensation as you hold, and then let go (*key word*). Repeat.

14. Squeeze your buttocks together as tight as you can. Hold them in this position, and then relax (*key word*). Repeat.

15. Pull your stomach in as far as you can. Feel the tightness of your abdominal muscles. Hold this position and then let go (*key word*). Repeat.

16. Now take the next two minutes to continue to relax, becoming more and more at ease, lighter and lighter, so light you feel as if you are floating. Then, counting backward from five to one, slowly "awaken." Open your eyes and sit up. You should be fully alert and completely relaxed.

After you have practiced your relaxation exercises for a week, you can reduce the number of steps by combining exercises for different muscle groups together. This will decrease the number of steps from 16 to 8:

- Eliminate step 1 (breathing)
- Combine steps 2 and 4 (clenching fists and shrugging shoulders)
- Combine steps 3 and 5 (bending arms and arching back)
- Combine steps 6 and 8 (pointing toes and chin to chest)
- Combine steps 7 and 9 (flexing toes and head back)
- Combine steps 10 and 12 (raising eyebrows and wide mouth)
- Combine steps 11 and 13 (lips tight and eyelids squeezed shut)
- Combine steps 14 and 15 (buttocks and stomach)
- Do step 16 by itself—do not combine it with any other step

Use the eight-step approach for another week, once a day (the exercises should now only take about ten minutes).

It is essential that you practice your relaxation exercises on a regular basis and for the prescribed period of time. If you do this, after two weeks you will have developed the skill of deep muscle relaxation. Then it's time to apply it to situations you encounter every day.

The final phase of relaxation training involves using what you have learned in real-life situations. To do this requires two steps. First, you need to identify feelings of tension in your body. Second, you need to replace these feelings with a state of relaxation.

Identifying feelings of tension in your body should be easy. For two weeks you have tensed your muscles and concentrated on how this feels. But replacing the tense feelings with relaxation will require something new. Because it's not always feasible to lie down and do the exercises (even the eight-step approach) when in the middle of an activity, you will need to bring on the feelings you had when relaxing your muscles during your exercises without actually doing the exercises. This is done by using your key word ("calm," "relax," or "let go") and then concentrating on releasing tension from wherever it is located in your body.

To do this effectively takes some practice. At first, try it in situations that are only a little anxiety producing. Later on, as you become accustomed to using this technique, you can apply it in more stressful circumstances.

Jennifer, a patient of mine, found deep muscle relaxation to be very helpful for managing anxiety in social situations. She used to get extremely tense at social functions where she did not know many people.

In response to her tension, Jennifer would eat nonstop at social events. At parties she would position herself next to the buffet table. When dining out with other people, she would lose control and consume everything in sight.

After she became good at using the eight-step version of the deep muscle technique, Jennifer began applying relaxation, using her key word, at parties and other social gatherings. She began with situations that made her a little uneasy. After successfully using her new skill in these situations, she tried more difficult ones.

Today Jennifer no longer uses food to deal with social anxiety. Instead she gets rid of the tension by substituting relaxation. You can do this too!

Abdominal Breathing

While deep muscle relaxation focuses on releasing muscle tension, abdominal breathing concentrates on changing breathing patterns.

When people are nervous, their breathing becomes shallow and rapid. This can result in not enough oxygen being supplied to the brain. In its extreme, this type of breathing can end up in hyperventilation, which can cause you to feel dizzy and light-headed.

Abdominal breathing, sometimes referred to as diaphragmatic breathing, teaches you how to breathe deeply, that is, from your diaphragm. Breathing in this way invokes feelings of calmness and relaxation.

The procedure is done as follows:

1. First place your hand on your abdomen (the part of your stomach that is below your waist).
2. Now inhale slowly and deeply, all the way down to where your hand is resting. If done correctly, you will feel your stomach push out.
3. Hold the breath for three seconds and then exhale slowly. Use your key word from your deep muscle relaxation exercises ("relax," "let go," or "calm") as you exhale.
4. Do a total of ten complete (inhale and exhale) breaths. You may find it helpful to count for each part of the exercise: inhale—one…two…three, hold—one…two…three, exhale —one…two…three. This will help you develop a slow, smooth rhythm.

Abdominal breathing only takes a few minutes to do. Practice it once a day for a couple of weeks, and then try using it when you begin to feel those uptight sensations in your body.

You now have two different techniques for reducing the physical feelings of anxiety. Whether you use one or both relaxation methods doesn't matter. What matters is that you consistently apply a relaxation procedure when you first become aware of tense feelings in your body. In this way you will eliminate the anxiety and the unnecessary eating that it triggers.

By using your relaxation procedures, your eating patterns will change. You no longer will go to the vending machine when you get tense over a project at work. You won't stand in front of the refrigerator snacking when your kids are being difficult. When you're out to dinner with strangers, you'll eat one piece of bread rather than the whole bread basket. Since the anxiety will be replaced with relaxation, your emotional trigger for overeating will be gone.

CHANGING ANXIOUS THINKING

People are *always* thinking. Often we are not aware of our thoughts, but they are always there.

Thoughts reflect feelings. When we are nervous, our thoughts are upsetting. Thoughts not only mirror nervous feelings, but once they occur they further increase our level of anxiety.

For example, let's suppose you are going to give a talk during a PTA meeting at your child's school. You feel nervous. You think, "What if I forget what I was going to say?" After you have this thought you're even more nervous than before.

Or you're having some people over to your home for the first time. You're a little tense. You think, "What if they don't like me?" Then you feel even more anxious about their visit.

That's the way anxious thinking works. While at first it reflects the overaroused state of our bodies, it then escalates us to even higher levels of tension.

Because of the role thoughts play in feelings and in triggering overeating, it is very important to eliminate those that are anxiety producing. To do this, you can use two different techniques for changing your thoughts, coping self-statements and thought-stopping.

"What-If" Anxiety

The upsetting thoughts we have when we are nervous come on very suddenly and unexpectedly. For this reason, we will refer to them as "automatic" thoughts.

The automatic thoughts of anxious people usually revolve around the themes of danger and an inability to cope. The likelihood of danger or threat in situations is overestimated or magnified, while the perception of ability to handle problems is underestimated or minimized.

Automatic thoughts often are "what-if" thoughts: "What if I get nervous and can't give the speech?" "What if the check doesn't arrive on time?" "What if I don't finish this project on time?" "What if I can't handle this?" "What if they don't like me?"

This type of thinking is your enemy. These thoughts lead you to assume the worst is going to happen and that you won't be able to deal with it when it does. While this is going on your anxiety skyrockets. And you, like all anxiety-triggered overeaters, end up eating.

Doris was an anxious overeater with whom I worked a few years ago. Doris was the queen of "what-if" thinking. Her worries permeated all aspects of her life—her relationship with husband, her performance on the job, her recreational activities, and her friendships.

She was constantly concerned that bad things were going to happen—her husband would get in a car accident, her friend would take something she said the wrong way and be hurt, she wouldn't get a project finished on deadline at the office and would be fired.

Doris's thinking was ruining her life. Her negative thoughts were creating overwhelming anxiety for her. And she was using food to try to cope with the feelings.

Through a lot of hard work, Doris eventually changed her thinking and took charge of her anxiety and her eating. You, too, can get rid of anxiety-producing thoughts. But first you need to be able to identify these thoughts as they are happening.

Identifying Your Anxious Thoughts

To get at the specific types of anxiety-producing thoughts you are having, you need to list your thoughts in the face of actual, real-life stresses. To do this, during or immediately after you have encountered a stressful or upsetting situation, write your thoughts down on a piece of paper. Do this for several different types of stressful situations, for a period of at least a few days.

Once you have your thought lists, go through them one by one.

Are there stresses that come up over and over again? Do your anxious thoughts tend to involve the same issues—your job, your children, your marriage, your finances? Do you exaggerate the potential negative consequences of your actions? Do you downplay your ability to meet challenges?

Terry came in with lists of her thoughts. When we went over them together, we found that certain thoughts that were related to the same themes kept reappearing.

Terry grew up in a very dysfunctional family. Her father, an alcoholic, was explosive and unpredictable, and was both physically and verbally abusive to her. When she was a child and adolescent, her father would repeatedly say to her, "You're stupid," "you can't do anything right," and "you won't amount to anything."

Even though she is now thirty-five, Terry still hears these comments in her head. When she faces a challenging situation at her job, her thoughts are remarkably similar to the things her father used to say to her. She thinks, "I won't be able to handle this...I'll fail and lose my job." After having these thoughts, Terry gets nervous and upset. She then, of course, eats to reduce the anxiety.

Terry's negative thoughts are not based on reality. She consistently gets excellent ratings from her supervisor and was recently promoted.

Terry is a good example of how unproductive and unrealistic our thinking can be. She is creating anxiety for herself through her irrational and negative thoughts. When she learns how to get rid of these thoughts by replacing them with coping self-statements, she will no longer overeat in response to them; the anxiety will disappear along with the thoughts.

Using Coping Self-Statements

Once you become aware of your anxious thoughts, you need to change them to more productive thoughts that encourage coping behavior. Changing your anxiety-producing thoughts to coping self-statements involves replacing the negative thoughts as they are occurring with positive thoughts. In other words, as soon as you notice that you are engaging in negative or "what-if" thinking, you immediately must switch to self-statements that focus on your ability to handle the situation.

In order to make the switch, you need to be armed with the new thoughts you will use. Make a list of positive alternatives to your negative thoughts—your coping self-statements—so that you can have them ready when you need them. The new thoughts should counter the negative thought.

Using the form on the next page, list your five most frequent anxiety-producing thoughts on the left (use the thought lists you made to do this). Then on the right side, directly opposite each thought, write down a positive alternative, that is, a coping self-statement that combats the idea expressed in the negative thought.

For example, if your negative thought is "I'm not getting this done fast enough," you can oppose this thought with the positive alternative, "If I take this step by step it will get done." If you think, "I'll never be successful at losing weight," you can replace this thought with, "I've been successful at other things, there's no reason I can't do this too." If you have the thought, "He won't like me," you can use the counterthought, "I'm a likable person" or "Who cares?"

Developing Coping Self-Statements

Negative Thoughts	Positive Alternatives (Coping Self-Statements)
1. _____	1. _____
2. _____	2. _____
3. _____	3. _____
4. _____	4. _____
5. _____	5. _____

Only you can come up with the coping self-statements that will work best for you. However, here are a few guidelines that will be helpful for generating your list:

1. Use "I" when creating your coping self-statements.
2. Do not use negatives. For instance, instead of saying, "I'm not going to get upset about this," say, "I can handle this."
3. Use words that are your own. For example, if you tend to refer to your boss as "the tyrant," use this phrase in your coping self-statement ("I can handle the tyrant").

Use your new coping self-statements whenever you find the negative and "what-if" thoughts cropping up. Since you are learning to break a bad habit you have most probably had for many years, this will take practice.

At first you may not actually believe your coping self-statements. This is not important. What matters is that you use them consistently to replace your negative automatic thoughts. Eventually, with time, you will come to believe the new thoughts that you are saying to yourself.

A tremendous amount of research has shown that coping self-statements effectively change people's moods. For anxiety (and depression, too—see chapter 6), this technique has consistently produced excellent results.

People frequently report that the effectiveness of coping self-statements is especially great when they come upon a particular self-statement that they can really relate to. You may also find this to be the case, as you continue to use this technique over time.

The payoff for changing your thinking is tremendous. You no longer will be creating undue anxiety for yourself (there's enough stress in life without you making things worse!). Becoming the master of your thoughts rather than their slave will decrease your anxiety and reduce your overeating.

Thought-Stopping

Although using coping self-statements is extremely effective for changing negative, anxiety-producing thoughts into positive thoughts, sometimes thinking gets really out of control and requires a different approach.

Obsessing occurs when we go on and on about a subject for a long period of time, getting ourselves more and more upset.

Obsessing is different from being preoccupied with something. Preoccupation does not bring on the intense emotions that accompany obsessing. And when you are preoccupied you usually are problem solving.

By contrast, obsessing about something does not help solve problems. What it does is cause spiraling levels of anxiety. For this reason, it must be cut off at its very start.

Let's take a look at two people who have problems with obsessing:

Ben has a high-pressure job. As a trial lawyer, he gets paid a lot of money for his services and is expected to give 110 percent effort to his clients. When he finishes his work for the day, Ben finds that he can't stop thinking about his cases. He replays meetings and telephone conversations he had that day, going over them again and again. He's worried that he might have said or done the wrong thing.

Although repeatedly reliving these events doesn't change anything that's happened, Ben's evening ritual does have a major effect on his life. He becomes more and more tense and anxious, and ends up eating to reduce the anxiety.

Nicole, like Ben, also does a lot of ruminating. Her obsessing starts after she has eaten something she feels she shouldn't have.

Nicole desperately wants to lose weight. Her family doctor has given her a diet. When she eats food that's not on the diet plan, she begins to think, "I can't believe I ate that...I'll never lose the weight...I have no self-control...I hate myself." This obsessing gets her extremely upset and—guess what—she then eats even more.

Thought-stopping is an extremely effective way to eliminate obsessing. The procedure was originally developed for people with obsessive-compulsive disorder, but works just as well for anyone who has difficulty cutting off upsetting thoughts. By getting rid of the ruminations, you will also get rid of the overeating they trigger. It worked for Ben and Nicole, and it will work for you.

The technique is easy to use. The only material you need to do this is a rubber band.

1. Place the rubber band on your left wrist (right wrist if you are left-handed).
2. As soon as you notice that you are obsessing about something, snap the rubber band (pull it away from your wrist with your free hand and then let it retract, hitting your wrist).
3. At the same time that you are snapping the rubber band, shout "STOP!" out loud. If you are in a place where you can't shout out loud, either whisper "stop!" or say it to yourself, in your head.

That's all there is to thought-stopping. The trick is to catch the obsessing sooner rather than later, so that you are able to cut it off early enough to avoid the anxiety-producing spiral that inevitably occurs.

Use the thought-stopping method religiously every single time you notice you are ruminating. At first you may find you have to repeat the procedure several times in a row to get rid of a single obsession. Eventually this won't be the case; you'll only need to do it once.

At first, wear the rubber band all the time. Later, as you progress, you can discontinue using it and just use the word *stop*.

Changing your thinking using coping self-statements and thought-stopping requires practice and diligence. However, your efforts will be repaid tenfold. Using these techniques will help you to decrease your anxiety and the eating it triggers.

GETTING RID OF FEARFUL BEHAVIOR

Anxious people usually have lots of fears. Because they have overactive autonomic nervous systems, they are prone to develop fearful reactions to objects, situations, and events that are (irrationally) perceived as potentially harmful.

While some people will "tough it out" when confronted with something they fear, many others completely avoid these situations. Avoidance is a very common and easy way to circumvent the discomfort that comes from facing fears (it also is a way that some people deal with their problems—see chapter 5 on the Avoider).

For example, let's assume you are afraid of public speaking. In order to circumvent the anxiety this brings on, you make sure you don't have to speak in public. You may turn down a job that offers more money but involves giving speeches. If you are in school, you may avoid taking classes that require you to make a presentation in front of the other students.

While avoiding situations that cause fear may work in the short run, it's not effective in the long run. That's because new situations keep coming up, meaning you will have to deal with the sudden surge of anxiety and figure a way out of the situation.

While you are thinking about how to escape situations that frighten you, you're eating. Like any other anxious overeater, you are using food to try to fight off the anxiety.

Beth is a good example of how fear leads to overeating. She is frightened of driving on highways. She always takes local streets to get where she needs to go, even if it takes her twice as long to get there.

Today Beth's mother is flying in to see her. Beth usually takes the back roads to get to the airport, but she's running late because she had to take her daughter to the doctor. If she takes her usual route, Beth will be half an hour late to meet her mother. She's afraid she'll panic if she takes the highway, which will get her there with time to spare.

While she's tormenting herself about what to do, Beth is shoving pretzels into her mouth. She's not hungry, she's nervous. And when she's nervous, she doesn't think about her weight or the consequences of overeating—she just wants to get rid of the anxiety.

It is not difficult to overcome fears. In doing so you no longer will have to come up with excuses and elaborate strategies to avoid things that make you uncomfortable. And you no longer will overeat because of the anxiety produced by these situations, because they won't make you anxious anymore.

The psychological technique that is used to combat fears is called *exposure*. The procedure involves very gradually and repeatedly confronting things (objects, events, places, people) that are avoided because of the anxiety they trigger.

Before we get to how to do the technique, you need to identify your particular fears, using the Fear Questionnaire below.

Fear Questionnaire

How often do you avoid the following because of nervous or scary feelings?

	Never	Sometimes	Often
1. Speaking in public	___	___	___
2. Small animals (dogs, cats)	___	___	___
3. Routine medical or dental procedures	___	___	___
4. Traveling away from home	___	___	___
5. Social gatherings	___	___	___
6. Elevators or escalators	___	___	___
7. Airplanes	___	___	___
8. Heights	___	___	___
9. Being alone	___	___	___
10. Driving on bridges, through tunnels, or on major highways	___	___	___
Other (describe): _____	___	___	___

Now take a look at those items you rated as "sometimes" or "often" on the questionnaire. These are the situations that are problematic for you, the ones that will benefit from exposure. (*Note:* For situations that make you nervous, but you don't avoid, you should use your relaxation and thought procedures to reduce anxiety. Exposure is only for anxiety-producing situations that you avoid.)

One Step at a Time

To use exposure you first need to break your fear down into pieces. This is done by developing a list of specific situations that are difficult for you, starting with those that produce only a small amount of fear, and then progressing up to those that trigger a lot of fear.

For example, Peggy has been fearful of taking elevators for the past ten years ever since she got stuck on one. Because of her fear, she "checks out" places she's planning on going to before actually getting there just to make sure she won't have to take an elevator.

In examining Peggy's fear, we found several factors that influenced her level of discomfort with elevators. Glass elevators, as opposed to the metal ones you can't see out of, were easier for her. Riding up one floor was less upsetting than riding up several floors. Having other people in the elevator with her was not as difficult as riding an elevator alone.

In coming up with a list of steps for exposure, Peggy and I used these three factors, combining different aspects of each of them, to arrive at situations that were easy, a little bit hard, hard, very hard, and "impossible."

Here are some of the items from Peggy's list:

Item:	Rating:
Taking a glass elevator with other people from the ground floor to the first floor	Easy
Taking a metal elevator with other people from the ground floor to the fifth floor	Hard
Taking a metal elevator alone from the ground floor to the tenth floor	Impossible

Peggy actually had ten steps on her list—these are only a few examples. Like Peggy, you will need to break your fear into ten items that range from easy to impossible.

Using the Fear Steps List on the next page, write down ten items in the column on the left side of the form. The first item on your list (number 1) should be your easiest situation, number 2 the next easiest one, and so on, until you reach number 10, which is the most difficult item.

Fear Steps List

Item   **Rating: 1–5**

1. _____   _____
2. _____   _____
3. _____   _____
4. _____   _____
5. _____   _____
6. _____   _____
7. _____   _____
8. _____   _____
9. _____   _____
10. _____   _____

Then, on the right side of the form, across from each item, give each situation a numerical rating from 1 to 5:

1 = *Easy*   no anxiety, don't avoid situation at all

2 = *Little hard*   a little anxiety, avoid situation occasionally

3 = *Hard*   definite anxiety, avoid situation frequently

4 = *Very hard*   severe anxiety, avoid situation almost all of the time

5 = *Impossible* overwhelming anxiety, avoid situation all of the time

Once you have your list you can begin the exposure exercises.

Confronting Your Fears

The effectiveness of exposure has been well documented in scientific literature. Although there has been some controversy as to the actual process by which this technique works, the overall consensus supports the notion that it deconditions fears that have been previously learned.

The procedure is done by having direct, face-to-face contact with the feared situation. This can sound pretty frightening. Nobody looks forward to doing things that make them uncomfortable.

However, by starting with steps that are only a little bit anxiety producing, and then *very slowly* moving on to more difficult steps, you will experience a minimum of discomfort.

Remember, once you have conquered your fear you will no longer need to deal with the anxiety that comes from trying to get out of situations—the very same anxiety that is causing you to overeat.

To implement the exposure technique, use your Fear Steps List and follow these instructions:

1. Face the object or situation that is described in item 1 until it no longer produces any anxiety or discomfort. Whether it takes one minute or one hour, stay in the situation until you feel OK. *Do not leave prematurely!*
2. Do step number 1 for the second item on your list.
3. Follow the same procedure for all of the remaining items on your list, doing them one at a time, progressing from the easiest to the hardest.

Tackle only one item from your list on any given day. It's best if you can do each item twice, on two different days, before moving on to the next one on your list. Your relaxation and thought techniques can be used to help you get through the exposure exercises.

To see how effective this technique is for conquering fears, meet Ellen, who overcame her fear with exposure.

When I first met Ellen she was terrified of dogs, even puppies. She had been this way since childhood, believing she had gotten this fear from her mother, who had the same problem.

Ellen's fear was affecting many aspects of her life. She was afraid to walk on the street because she might run into a dog. She was afraid to go to people's homes she hadn't been to before because they might have a dog. She completely avoided parks because dog owners and their pets were likely to be there.

Ellen did a lot of eating as a result of her fear. For instance, if she received a telephone call from a friend inviting her to a party at someone else's home, she immediately worried that there might be a dog there. Her anxiety then would shoot up and she would head for the refrigerator. If she was out to dinner on a first date, she would be concerned that her date would invite her back to his place after dinner. What if he had a dog—what would she do? While worrying about a potential dog encounter, Ellen devoured everything on the dinner table.

Ellen knew she had to do something about her anxiety. To begin she made up a list of her fears. She discovered that there were three factors related to her level of fear—the size of the dog, how close it was to her, and how active it was.

Ellen started off working on her fear by spending time with Jake, my toy poodle. Jake was the perfect dog for Ellen to begin with because he is extremely small (four pounds) and not too active.

At first Jake was kept on a leash, across the room from Ellen. Slowly, over the course of an hour, Jake got progressively closer to Ellen. By the end of the exposure session, Jake was off the leash and sitting on Ellen's lap!

Over the next few weeks Ellen confronted larger and more active dogs. Soon she was comfortable with virtually any dog. (I got a telephone call from Ellen about a year ago—she told me she had kept the weight off and had gotten a puppy!)

Exposure is an incredibly effective and permanent way to alleviate fears. Although it can be somewhat time consuming, the changes it makes are well worth the investment. As your fear dissipates so will your overeating. And then you will have what you always have wanted—a thin self, now and forever.

OTHER THINGS YOU SHOULD KNOW ABOUT

Caffeine, Alcohol, and Tobacco

Stress Reducers are notorious for using legal drugs (and sometimes the illegal type, too) to try to relax. However, use of caffeine, alcohol, and cigarettes is problematic, each for its own reasons.

Caffeine is a stimulant. *It increases anxiety!* More specifically, caffeine produces physiological effects on the body that are the same as those experienced when you are very nervous: increased heart rate, increased blood pressure, sweating, jitters, and headaches.

Since your goal is to learn how to reduce anxiety, ingesting caffeine products while in this program (and after this program) is counterproductive. You should make your best effort to reduce or completely eliminate caffeine.

Caffeine is found in large amounts in coffee, tea, chocolate, and many soft drinks. Check labels and become knowledgeable about which foods and drinks contain caffeine. Then work on replacing them with caffeine-free alternatives.

Stress Reducers often use (and sometimes abuse) alcohol. This is because alcohol, a depressant, is an easy way to get rid of the tension and worry that come with anxiety.

Besides possible health problems associated with overuse of alcohol, drinking can undermine the effectiveness of this program. Alcohol stands in the way of learning true coping strategies for dealing with stress.

During this program and afterward, please try to reduce or completely eliminate your intake of alcoholic beverages. I know at first this may be hard, but trust me, it will be worth it!

Tobacco products, particularly cigarettes, frequently are used by Stress Reducers to help them relax. Nicotine is a biphasic drug; it is capable of producing two different types of effects. In people who smoke regularly (two or fewer packs a day), the effect is usually that of a stimulant (in contrast, chain smokers may experience a relaxation effect from the drug). In other words nicotine is actually *increasing* their anxiety level, not reducing it.

A second problem with nicotine is that smokers repeatedly go through mini episodes of nicotine withdrawal between cigarettes. This produces anxiety as well and is what motivates smokers to head for another fix of the drug.

While most cigarette smokers swear that cigarettes relax them, physiologically this is simply not the case (except, perhaps, if you are a chain smoker). You *think* it relaxes you because you feel better when you alleviate the anxiety accompanying withdrawal following a period of abstinence.

If you are a smoker and a Stress Reducer, you should be aware that you are actually making yourself more tense by smoking. This will make following your treatment program for overeating some-what more difficult.

The anxiety-reduction techniques you are now using to eliminate your overeating will work for your smoking. This is one case where you might want to consider tackling two problems at once—your smoking and your weight—because the same treatment techniques will work for both problems.

Blood Sugar, Anxiety, and Overeating

When the level of sugar in your blood drops you become irritable, tense, and jittery. If you are a Stress Reducer, these type of symptoms, which closely resemble anxiety, lead you to overeat.

For this reason it is important to keep your blood-sugar level as steady and even as possible. The best way to do this is to eat on a regular basis, at least three well-spaced meals a day, or, better yet, four to six smaller meals a day.

It is also a good idea to avoid certain types of foods that trigger substantial swings in your blood-sugar level—for example, processed sugar. Although sugar products initially give you a burst of energy, they let you down just as suddenly. With your blood-sugar level depleted, you feel anxious, and the urge to overeat is overwhelming.

Premenopausal women may find that their anxiety level and eating increase the week prior to menstruation. It is especially important to pay attention to your blood-sugar level during this time. Also, some of the tension you experience before your period can be reduced by decreasing water retention and bloating: Avoid excessive use of salt and sodium-rich foods, drink plenty of water, and eat naturally diuretic foods that increase urine flow, such as grapefruit and cranberry juice.

AFTER COMPLETING THE PROGRAM

Stress Reducers respond to stress and anxiety by eating. Because anxiety is at the root of their weight problem, diets, which focus on food, are not effective for them. If you're an anxiety-triggered overeater, the only way to maintain lifelong weight control is to directly attack the underlying cause of the overeating—anxiety.

During the five weeks of this program you will have learned a variety of anxiety-reduction methods. But your job is not finished. You need to continue to apply these techniques in your everyday life, and not just for a few months, but forever.

As a person who always (since childhood) has been prone to tension, I have used these psychological tools for the past twenty-two years. This is not a chore—it is a pleasure! Not only have I kept my weight down during this period, but I feel terrific.

Over time your new skills will become habits—very good ones. You won't have to consciously apply them every time you get uptight. You will come to use them automatically, without paying much attention to them. That's when you know you really have reached your goal.

Stress Reducers benefit from using the anxiety-reduction methods in all areas of their life, not only in maintaining control of their weight. Eliminating excess tension and learning how to relax will have positive effects on everything you do—your relationships, your job, your recreational activities—and on how you feel about yourself.

With these treatment methods, practice, and patience, you will become the thin person you have always dreamed of. Your fantasy-self finally will become your real self! And not just for now, but for all the years that are to come.

5

The Avoider:
Taking Care of Business

Ellen has been in the same job for eight years. When she first got her master's degree in business, she had high hopes for an exciting, fulfilling career. But as the years have gone by she has been passed over for the really good opportunities, overshot by more assertive and outgoing employees who have successfully worked their way up the corporate ladder.

Shy by nature and lacking the confidence to confront her superiors, Ellen has resorted to eating as a way of avoiding dealing with the realities of her situation. Unhappy in her present position but unable to do anything about it, she escapes thinking about her situation through food.

As you discovered in chapter 1, Avoiders eat to escape dealing with life's problems. Eating is used as an avoidance strategy, so that problems can be put "on hold," rather than confronted and solved.

Some Avoiders eat to escape making major life decisions, such as career or marriage choices, while others use food to avoid facing (and potentially rectifying) poor choices that they have already made (a failing marriage, a dead-end job).

Sometimes the problem is an old hurt or trauma that can't be faced. As an example of this, Oprah Winfrey, on her television program and in her other media appearances, has spoken about the role of childhood abuse in the development of her own eating problem. Apparently, her inability to face and deal with these traumatic early experiences resulted in overeating and obesity.

Rather than facing and solving problems, the Avoider buries his or her head in the sand, or, in this case, in the refrigerator. By not confronting problems head-on, the Avoider ensures that the problems will continue, and then eats in response. In this way, avoiding problems and eating become a vicious cycle—eating to avoid dealing with a problem, causing the problem to continue because it has not been dealt with, which causes eating again because of the problem, and so on.

The solution, of course, is to confront and solve the problem rather than continuing to avoid it. By doing this, you will find the need for overeating disappears.

But before we get into the specifics of the treatment approach for the Avoider, let's look at some of the factors that lead to the development of this eating profile.

THE CAUSES OF AVOIDANT EATING

Why do people use food to escape their problems? I believe the answer is, in many ways, the same as for drugs and alcohol.

When you use substances instead of facing a problem, the problem ends up being put on hold. By not dealing with the problem, you do not experience the discomfort or upset that comes with facing the situation.

So, in a sense, eating "works"—it gets you out of or away from a bad situation and makes you feel temporarily better. The downside to this, of course, is that you keep getting larger. And because the problem that is triggering your eating has not gone away, you wind up with two problems—the original difficulty and your weight problem.

By and large, using food as an avoidance strategy is a learned behavior.

How do we learn it? Through several means. First is the influence of our parents. When many of us were children, if we were upset, if things were not going well, or if there was a problem that we were facing, our parents directed us to food. Although they may have had the best of intentions, the end result was often very problematic. With enough repetition, one can easily get into the habit of turning to food when confronted by upsetting feelings and problems.

Our parents also influence us through our observation and imitation of their behavior. As children, we often end up first imitating, then permanently adopting, the behaviors displayed by our parents. Did you frequently observe family members turning to food when faced with problems? Did your mother or father use eating as an avoidance strategy?

There also are other influences around us, besides our families, that play a role in how we approach dealing with conflicts and problems.

In the eighties there was a very popular show on television called *Dallas*. One of the things that I remember most about that show was how almost every one of the characters in it went for a drink whenever there was a problem (and there were a lot of problems on that show—it was the first prime-time soap opera). Someone said something upsetting to Sue Ann—she poured herself a drink. J.R.'s business deal didn't go well—he went to the local bar.

In the forties and fifties you saw the same type of behavior displayed in movies, but with cigarettes. When Bogie and Bergman had to decide what to do about their relationship in *Casablanca*, they reached for their cigarettes. Ditto Lauren Bacall, Kate Hepburn, and Spencer Tracy.

Fortunately, in the last decade we have seen a decrease in the depiction of drinking and smoking in television and movies as the popularity of using these substances has declined. However, for those of us who were brought up in the forties, fifties, sixties, and seventies, the idea of escaping problems with substances is old hat, and, unfortunately, a style we too often adopted.

Another entirely different risk factor for becoming an Avoider is gender. Females are more likely than males to use food in avoiding their problems. This probably is because females are less likely to have the assertiveness and problem-solving skills needed to effectively confront problems.

This is not to say that women cannot develop these skills—they certainly have the ability to do so, as many women have proven. However, society sends mixed signals to females regarding the value of these attributes for them. Assertiveness, while considered a positive trait for men, sometimes is viewed differently for women who are labeled bossy, difficult, demanding, or loud.

As a corollary to this, many married women believe that it is their husband's job to handle the difficulties that come up in life. Oftentimes, these are woman who went from being taken care of by their parents to being taken care of by their husbands, never really learning how to take care of themselves.

While confronting the realities of the business world is a good teacher of survival skills, some women never take part in the workplace, opting to focus exclusively on raising a family. Certainly there are a great many female homemakers who have excellent problem-solving skills. But for others, it may be hard to learn the adult management of problems if they haven't already picked up these skills before marriage and children.

THE PSYCHOLOGICAL APPROACH TO AVOIDANT EATING

The Avoider uses food to avoid dealing with life's problems. Rather than identifying and confronting problems directly, they escape or avoid their difficulties through eating.

If you are an Avoider and you want to get permanent control over your eating you must adopt a new strategy for dealing with your problems. By developing skills to effectively handle your problems you will no longer run to food. You will become confident and assertive, managing the variety of troubles that you need to deal with during your lifetime.

In this program, first you will learn how to correctly identify your emotions, facing and accurately labeling your feelings so that you can begin to get a handle on your problems. Next, you will develop problem-solving and assertiveness skills, so that you can come up with solutions to your problems and then put those solutions to work. Finally, we will cover the technique of visualization, where you can try out and practice your new strategies in your imagination.

Program for the Avoider

Treatment Method	Begin
Identifying emotions	Week 1
Problem-solving skills	Week 2
Assertiveness training	Week 3
Visualization	Week 4

FACING YOUR FEELINGS

Avoiders are notorious for being in the dark about their own emotions. They either have no clue as to how they are feeling, or inaccurately label their emotions (e.g., mistaking anger for anxiety).

Being unaware of their true feelings serves an important purpose for Avoiders—it enables them to avoid confronting whatever problems are facing them. If you don't acknowledge that something is wrong, you certainly can't be expected to take actions to correct the problem.

Correctly identifying and labeling your emotions is a necessary component to all effective problem solving. Here we are particularly concerned with your negative feelings. These are the emotions that alert you to the fact that something isn't going right, that there is a problem.

Stacy is a good example of an Avoider who had a problem acknowledging her negative feelings.

When I first met Stacy, one of the things I asked her about was her marriage. Although her response at that time was "Great," I later found out that her husband had been unfaithful to her for many years.

Although Stacy had found enough clues to strongly suggest that her husband had been cheating, two plus two did not equal four for her. Whenever she felt upset or concerned about her husband, she buried her head in the sand—in this case, pizza, potato chips, cookies, and the like. Rather than facing her feelings and discovering the truth, she insisted to herself and to others that her marriage was fine. By avoiding facing reality, she didn't have to think about the possibility of divorce and how she might survive on her own. Stacy "solved" her problem by denying its existence.

Unfortunately, while she was doing this, her weight ballooned upward. Each year she gained 10 to 20 pounds until she leveled off at 210.

If you are an Avoider the first step in taking control of your eating problem is to learn to accurately identify your feelings, particularly the negative ones. Whether you are avoiding facing a current relationship problem like Stacy, or a deep hurt from the past, you will not be able to solve the situation and stop overeating without first acknowledging how you feel.

Daily Food Record

Date: _____

Time	Meal or Snack?	Planned?	Emotion Preceding Eating

In all likelihood, much of your snacking and overeating occurs immediately following a negative emotion. Monitoring the feelings you have before you eat is a good first step toward attending to and correctly identifying emotions.

Make photocopies of the Daily Food Record on page 102. Record the emotions that you have immediately prior to eating every day for at least a week. Remember to include all of your snacks as well as your meals. Identifying the feelings that precede unplanned eating (e.g., the candy bar you unexpectedly "give in to" in the afternoon) will be particularly useful.

In filling in the last column on the form, "emotion preceding eating," you may find it helpful to refer to the following list, particularly if you have trouble identifying how you feel.

Negative Emotions

Angry, mad, furious
Hurt, upset, wounded
Sad, depressed, unhappy
Bored, lonely, empty

Nervous, worried, fearful
Jealous, envious, resentful
Ashamed, embarrassed,
  mortified

Positive Emotions

Happy, joyful, cheerful
Excited, thrilled, elated
Content, pleased, comfortable

Energetic, alive, vital
Relaxed, quiet, peaceful

It is possible that you may notice a change in your eating habits just by doing the monitoring. By paying attention to the emotions (particularly the negative ones) that you experience before you eat, you may be alerted to problems that require your attention. If your response is to deal with the problem at hand rather than head for the refrigerator, your overeating will subside and you will lose weight.

Most Avoiders, however, do not possess the skills needed to effectively confront their problems. Although monitoring may alert them to their negative feelings, they do not know what to do from there. For them, acknowledging how they feel is an important and critical first step, but is not sufficient in and of itself to produce behavior change.

So, now that you know how you feel, what do you do with the

feelings? Because negative feelings are almost always uncomfortable, you will be motivated to get rid of them. Unfortunately, since you are in the habit of using food to solve, or, rather, not solve, your problems, you may be tempted to eat in response to these uncomfortable feelings. This is exactly what you should not do! Instead, you need to use the feeling, once identified, as the first clue in helping you decipher what is wrong or what the problem is. You will have to use your negative feelings, even embrace them, as an important source of information.

Think of yourself as a detective following clues to unravel a mystery. In pursuing the mystery, your feelings are important indicators as to what is going on.

If you eat when you have an unpleasant feeling you will not become an effective problem solver. Eating will distract you from the issue at hand and make you (at least, temporarily) feel better. Consequently, you will lose your motivation to identify and solve your problems.

DEVELOPING PROBLEM-SOLVING ABILITIES

There are four steps to problem solving. The first step is to identify the problem. As discussed earlier, your feelings should serve as an early warning signal that a problem is at hand.

When you have an unpleasant feeling the first question you need to ask yourself is "What exactly am I feeling?" Once you have identified the emotion, your second, immediate question needs to be "Why am I feeling this way?" This is how you will begin to figure out what the problem is.

To determine why you are experiencing a negative emotion at a particular point in time, you need to look both inside (your thoughts) and outside (your surroundings) yourself.

As mentioned in chapter 4, although we are thinking virtually all of the time we seldom are aware of our thoughts. But our thoughts, whether conscious or not, exert a powerful influence over our feelings. Our thoughts alone can trigger any of the negative (or positive) feelings that we experience.

To be able to identify problems relies, at least to some extent, on being aware of your thoughts. When you have a negative feeling and the reason is not readily apparent, you need to immediately scan your thoughts. You need to ask yourself, "What was I thinking about right before I started to have this feeling?"

Your feelings don't originate in a vacuum. Either something has happened in your environment or in your head, or both, to trigger the feeling that you are having. Your job, as detective, is to figure out which, and what, it is.

Getting into the habit of scanning your thoughts definitely takes practice. But the good news is that once you get it, you really have gotten it—scanning your thoughts becomes something you do automatically whenever you need it.

For most people, scanning your *environment* for clues as to why you are feeling a certain way is easier than scanning thoughts. You simply work on making a connection between environmental events—for example, a fight with your spouse—and your feelings.

Some problems, of course, are easier to identify than others. Problems that are difficult to identify usually are those that would cause us extreme discomfort or psychological pain to acknowledge. Our psyche usually develops a solid wall as a defense to protect us from experiencing this pain, and this can make it very difficult to get in touch with what really is troubling us.

In situations like this, your dreams can sometimes help point you in the right direction. If a particular upsetting theme keeps reappearing in your dreams it likely is representative of a psychological conflict that has not yet been resolved. Another way to get at hidden problems is through keeping a journal of your thoughts and feelings. Finally, psychotherapy helps many people to identify and understand hidden issues.

Although some problems are difficult to get at, most are fairly apparent, if you just look at the internal and external clues.

Take Beth, for example. Having worked as an elementary school teacher in the same school for almost ten years, Beth loved her work but despised the school's principal. He had caused Beth to suffer under his supervision by belittling her, minimizing her abilities, and undercutting her authority in her own classroom for way too long.

Although she was terribly unhappy, Beth was uncertain as to whether anyone else would want to hire her. Even if she did find another position, she was concerned about leaving the familiarity of her current job for the unknown. Compounding the problem was

Beth's fear that if she tried to get another job, and her principal found out she was looking, she might face negative consequences.

We will come back to Beth shortly, but, for now, let's continue with our discussion of problem solving.

THE FOUR STEPS OF PROBLEM SOLVING

STEP 1   Identify the problem, fully analyzing all facets of the situation

STEP 2   Identify a number of realistic, possible solutions

STEP 3   Evaluate each possible solution for likely outcome, and select one

STEP 4   Implement the chosen solution and evaluate outcome

After the problem has been identified, you need to determine whether it is a problem that you can do anything about. As I am sure you already know, there are some things we have control over and others we don't. It is the things that we can exert control over that will benefit from problem-solving skills.

If you are an Avoider, you most likely minimize the likelihood of having control over a solution. Your response to problems typically is "*Que sera sera*," or "I can't do anything about that."

While there certainly are situations that you can't do anything about—an upcoming storm, paying taxes—there are many other situations that will respond positively to the appropriate solutions.

After identifying the problem, assuming it is a problem that you can do something about, the second step of problem solving is to formulate several possible solutions to the problem.

Beth came up with one possible solution to her problem (look for another job) but subsequently thought of a variety of "reasons" why this solution wouldn't work. Let's consider whether there are any other possible answers to her problem.

Another potential solution to Beth's problem might be to confront the school principal about his unkind and unconstructive behavior. Alternatively, Beth could have considered going over his head, reporting his behavior to the school board. If legal issues were involved (for example, sexual harassment) she might have thought about filing a legal suit against him.

In coming up with possible solutions to a problem you need to be creative. The most obvious solution is not necessarily the only or the best option. Beth, for instance, thought that finding another job was the only possible answer to her problem. While this certainly was a reasonable solution, alternative solutions were not considered.

Spend a minute trying to identify at least one problem that you currently have, and then come up with at least three possible ways to address that problem.

When you come up with possible solutions to your problem, make sure they are feasible. For example, while winning the lottery might be the answer to your financial difficulties, the likelihood of this actually happening is minuscule.

The third step in problem solving involves evaluating each of the potential solutions you came up with. Solutions to problems differ on several levels:

Viability: How likely is it that you will be able to undertake this option? Do you have the ability or resources to put the plan into action?

Suitability: How well matched is this option to the problem? In other words, how well does it address the problem?

Consequences: What are the potential positive and negative outcomes from exerting this option, and how likely are they to occur?

Take a look at the first potential solution that you listed. Is it viable? Can you actually make it happen? What about suitability? Does the solution really take care of the problem? Is it only a "Band-Aid," or temporary fix? Does it address the whole problem, or just part of it?

If the solution is viable and suitable, your next job is to look at the pluses and minuses associated with that particular choice. What good things might happen if you exert this option? What bad things? What is the probability of each of these good and bad things happening?

Take each of the possible solutions that you outlined earlier and list the potential positive and negative consequences that may be associated with that option. Also, rate from 1 to 10 the likelihood of that consequence occurring.

Now compare your three different solutions. A solution that has a high likelihood of positive consequences while simultaneously having a low likelihood of negative consequences is the ideal solution. Unfortunately, very few solutions fall into this category.

In a less-than-perfect world, we may have to be satisfied with solutions that have relatively more positives and relatively fewer negatives compared to the other possible solutions on our list.

As an example of how this works, let's take a look at Stephanie. At forty-one, Stephanie has never been married. She desperately wants to have children and is concerned that her biological clock is running out.

Stephanie currently is dating two men. One, Tom, has asked her to marry him. A widower without children, he, like Stephanie, wants to have a family. The other man, Bart, is divorced and has joint custody of his two children. Bart says that he will never marry again and does not want any more children (he had a vasectomy immediately following his divorce).

Although Stephanie cares deeply about Tom, and thinks he would be a wonderful husband and father, she is concerned about a certain lack of passion between them. Her relationship with Bart, on the other hand, is just the opposite—exciting and intense.

Stephanie has a problem that does not have a perfect solution. Although she experiences "fireworks" with Bart, he does not share the same life goals (i.e., marriage and children) as she. On the other hand, if she marries Tom, she will probably have the family she desires, but may have to live with less passion than she would like.

After seriously evaluating her options, Stephanie ultimately decided to marry Tom. Today, years later, she has a five-year-old daughter, and is very happy with her relationship with Tom. (As an aside, Bart actually did end up getting married—to a woman twenty-five years his junior.)

After evaluating and choosing a solution, the final step in problem solving is to implement the solution you have chosen, and then evaluate its outcome. Implementing your solution often relies to some degree on the ability to assertively and effectively communicate with others, which is covered in detail in the next section of this chapter.

Evaluating the outcome of your solution—that is, observing the extent to which it worked—is your feedback on how well you did at solving a particular problem. In the continuing development of your problem-solving abilities, much is to be learned by honestly assessing the outcome of your attempts to confront problems. Through acknowledging your successes as well as your mistakes, you will become a better and more experienced problem solver.

DEVELOPING AN ASSERTIVE STYLE

Avoiders usually are people-pleasers. They do not want to rock the boat. They have a difficult time communicating their own needs and wants, concerned they may conflict with those of other people. They are extremely reluctant to express negative feelings or say no. Their goal is to be universally liked and to avoid conflict at all costs.

While a passive, pleasing communication style may be comfortable for those around you, it is not comfortable for you. Not expressing how you really feel leads most Avoiders to the refrigerator, where they attempt to distract and comfort themselves with food.

Moreover, it is not possible to put the solutions to most problems into action without assertiveness skills. Solving problems usually includes, at least in part, the ability to have direct, clear, and honest communications.

An assertive style differs substantially from an aggressive style. Aggressive people are hostile, rude, and demanding, showing no respect for the rights or needs of other people. By contrast, assertive people are direct and honest about their feelings, but, at the same time, demonstrate appropriate behavior toward others.

To understand better where you fall along the assertiveness continuum, complete the Assertiveness Questionnaire on page 112.

As you probably can guess, yes answers to these questions are indicative of an assertiveness problem. The greater the number of yes responses, the greater the difficulty you have with expressing yourself in an assertive manner.

Assertiveness includes both verbal and nonverbal behavior. Expressing yourself in a direct, honest, and clear way is one way that you get your point across. How you hold your body, your eye contact, tone of voice, and facial expression also contribute to how others perceive you, and how they will "read" your message.

Assertiveness Questionnaire

Answer yes or no to each of the following questions:

	Yes	No
1. Is it difficult or uncomfortable for you to return something at a store?	—	—
2. Do you have a hard time saying no to family or friends?	—	—
3. Is it difficult for you to ask for small favors from other people?	—	—
4. Is it hard for you to express how you really feel?	—	—
5. Is it hard for you to call attention to something you believe is unfair?	—	—
6. Is it difficult for you to call attention to another person's error?	—	—
7. Is it hard for you to ask for what you really want?	—	—
8. Are you generally uncomfortable with authority figures?	—	—
9. Are you reluctant to share your own ideas or to propose plans?	—	—
10. Do you have a hard time ending relationships that are unsatisfactory?		

Nonverbal Communication

Imagine going in to see your boss and asking for a raise. Although you might say the right things, your nonverbal behavior can send a message that is at odds with what you want to communicate. For instance, if your head is down, your shoulders slumped, and your eyes averted, you would not look like you really thought you deserved a raise, despite what you might be saying.

Let's start by focusing on the *nonverbal* skills you need to assertively communicate your thoughts and feelings.

Eye contact: Look directly, but respectfully (no glaring), into the eyes of the person you are communicating with.

Body language: Sit or stand straight up, with good posture and square shoulders. Maintain an "open" position (don't cross your arms or legs). You want your body language to suggest that you are relaxed and confident, not closed and rigid. If you are standing, keep both feet on the ground and do not back up or move away.

Tone of voice: Remain calm and do not get overly emotional; a calm, assertive statement is much more effective than an emotional outburst. Keep the tone of your voice level and even.

To work on these nonverbal assertiveness skills, try practicing them by role-playing with a friend or family member (someone you feel very comfortable with). You can use these skills in conjunction with verbal assertiveness skills in some of the practice situations described later on in this chapter.

Speaking Up for Yourself

Verbal assertiveness skills are somewhat more complex than nonverbal assertiveness skills. Verbal assertiveness deals, to a large extent, with the content of your communication. With content, judgment comes into play: What I may consider an assertive response may be viewed differently (as passive, or aggressive) by others. Verbal assertiveness, therefore, is less objective than nonverbal assertiveness, where it is easy to measure the presence or absence of key nonverbal behaviors (either you are looking at the person or you are not).

Despite these caveats, the general consensus is that assertive verbal responses include each of the following ingredients.

1. Clearly state your thoughts and feelings honestly, directly, and appropriately. Do not use sarcasm or blame. Begin your statement with an "I" rather than a "you", e.g., "I feel..." rather than "You..." Try to be brief.
2. State what you want, clearly and directly, e.g., "I want you to..." If necessary, repeat your message. Do not be side-tracked, do not participate in a debate or argument; stay solution oriented.
3. If appropriate, state the consequences (positive or negative) of getting or not getting what you requested in number 2, e.g., "If you do not refund my money I will need to speak with your supervisor." Do not be hostile or condescending; speak in a matter-of-fact tone of voice.

As you can see, the first step in developing an assertive response is to communicate your own thoughts or feelings, which you worked on earlier in this program. The second step, stating what you want, is where you try to implement your chosen solution, the one you picked following careful evaluation of multiple possible solutions. To briefly sum up the first two steps, first you are expressing the problem and then you are proposing a solution (often in the form of a request) to that problem.

For example, if you are having problems in your marriage you might say to your spouse, "I am unhappy with the way things have been going between us [statement of the problem]. I would like for us to go for marital counseling [proposing a solution to the problem]."

Another example would be asking your boss for a raise. An assertive approach might be, "Given my contributions to this company, I think that I am underpaid [statement of the problem]. I would like a ten percent raise beginning January first [proposing a solution to the problem]."

The third and final step of assertive communications involves stating the consequences for cooperating or not cooperating with the proposed solution. In our example of marital problems, this step might involve saying, "By going for marital counseling, I will know that you are committed to making our marriage work," or "I think that marriage counseling will really help us get back on the right track" (stating positive consequences).

In the raise example, the third step might be, "Getting this raise will let me know that you value my contribution to this company" (statement of positive consequences). However, if the boss seems reluctant to accept your proposed solution to the problem (that is, he or she does not appear willing to agree to a raise), you may want to express potential negative consequences for a failure to comply with your request: "If I do not get a raise I may have to look into employment opportunities elsewhere" (statement of negative consequences). Obviously, you only want to make this statement if you are ready and willing to follow this course of action.

It is not always necessary or appropriate to state consequences. For instance, if you go to return merchandise at a department store, you usually do not need to point out potential positive or negative consequences for the salesperson's cooperation. The decision to include a statement of consequences depends, to some degree, on the amount of resistance you anticipate or actually confront in a given individual.

Below are a few sample situations that you can use as exercises to practice your verbal assertiveness skills. First, write out your responses. Then, with the help of a friend or family member, role-play your assertive responses. Following this, you should be ready to start trying your new behaviors out in the real world.

You go out to lunch with a girlfriend. When the check arrives, you see that you have been overcharged by five dollars. You say to the server...

State the problem:

State the solution:

State the consequences (if appropriate):

You wash your new shirt according to the care instructions on the label. It comes out looking faded and worn. You take it back to the store where you bought it and address the salesclerk.

State the problem:

State the solution:

State the consequences (if appropriate):

You are in the nonsmoking section of a restaurant. The woman at the table next to you lights up a cigarette. You decide to speak up.

State the problem:

State the solution:

State the consequences (if appropriate):

Your fiancé has been spending more time with friends than with you. You are feeling neglected. You decide to discuss it with him (or her).

State the problem:

State the solution:

State the consequences (if appropriate):

Saying No

Saying no is a special case of assertiveness that is particularly rough for many Avoiders. In saying no, you may have to face the displeasure of the person you are turning down, a situation that is very uncomfortable for the people-pleasing Avoider.

Why is saying no so difficult to do? A lot of this has to do with the way we perceive this behavior. If you view saying no as a way of taking care of yourself, rather than a "bad" behavior that you should feel guilty about, it will be easier for you to do. Setting limits on what you will and will not do for other people is a way of showing self-respect.

When you say yes when you really want to say no, you end up eating in response to your internal conflict. Eating is your way of running away from the problem at hand. Face the problem, solve it, and you won't need to overeat.

How do you say no without choking on the word as it comes out of your mouth? Well, the way that you do this depends on the situation. If you want to say no to someone you don't have a relationship with, a simple "No, thank you" or "I'm not interested" should suffice. (If you are saying no in person, as opposed to on the telephone, make sure that your nonverbal behavior coincides with your verbal behavior.)

If you want to say no to a person with whom you have a relationship—a business acquaintance, family member, friend, etc.—it is usually best to offer an explanation as to why you are declining the request. Be honest and direct in offering your reason; then, if appropriate, you can offer an alternative that meets both of your needs.

For example, let's suppose your friend has scheduled an airplane flight for 6:00 A.M. on a weekday morning. She wants you to drive her to the airport before you go to work so that she won't have to leave her car in the airport parking lot for the two weeks she'll be away. You feel that getting up that early and then going to a full day of work is asking too much. You say, "I really think it would be very difficult for me to get up so early and then spend a full day at my office. If you can change it to an evening or weekend flight, I would be happy to take you."

You have given your friend an understandable and honest reason why you will not drive her to the airport, a reason for saying no. In addition, you offered a potential solution to the problem, one that would meet both of your needs.

But what if the person you are saying no to argues with you, giving you a hard time? The best thing to do in this situation is to simply repeat what you already have said, possibly raising your voice *slightly* (no yelling!) to show that your decision is final. Do *not* attempt to argue or expand your point, which may well lead to an escalation of the situation. Just firmly reiterate your point of view, and say no.

Assertiveness is the cornerstone of self-care. By looking out for yourself in this way, using these skills to effectively put your problem solutions into action, your eating will decrease. You will confront your difficulties head-on, rather than hiding from them with food.

PRACTICING YOUR NEW SKILLS WITH VISUALIZATION

The way to firm up your belief in your ability to solve problems and execute their solutions is to do just that: successfully confront them head-on. It is very hard, if not impossible, to change our view of our abilities without gathering evidence that we can do what we propose to do. That is why practice is so important for developing these new psychological skills.

While nothing quite substitutes for practice in the real world, it is helpful to practice in your own imagination either before or in addition to conducting real-life practice sessions. Having a chance to try out your new skills in your head before putting them to work in your daily life has two very positive aspects.

First, it affords a safe environment where you will not experience failure. It allows you to control the potential responses of those people you interact with, eliminating the possibility that other people will undermine your effectiveness. In other words, in your imagination, you are in complete control of the scenario—the event goes the way you want it to. This can be very helpful and encouraging, particularly early on in the building of new skills.

Second, visualization allows you to practice your new skills as often as you want—you don't have to wait for the right situation to pop up, as you frequently have to do in real life.

Practice visualizing yourself successfully tackling your problems. This will provide you with the practice and self-confidence you need to put your plans into action in real life.

1. In a quiet, comfortable place where you won't be interrupted, lie back and close your eyes.

2. Visualize yourself confronting and successfully dealing with a problem situation. Picture the situation as if it were a movie. To make the scene as real as possible, conjure up all of the sights, sounds, smells, and tastes that would accompany this situation. Picture the scene in your head for approximately two minutes.
3. Repeat the same scene again as many times as needed until you feel comfortable handling the situation.

OTHER THINGS YOU SHOULD KNOW ABOUT

Alcohol and the Avoider

Many Avoiders use alcohol in addition to overeating as a way to get out of dealing with their problems. Alcohol provides a brief mental reprieve from a problematic situation, and thus does not encourage problem-solving behavior—on the contrary, it actually interferes with the development of problem-solving skills because it puts your problem in a holding pattern.

If you often drink alcoholic beverages in the face of a problem, you must stop this as you embark on this program. Although it may be difficult to do this at the same time that you are working on your overeating, to learn the skills outlined in this chapter will require that you give up any and all substances that shield you from acknowledging your problems.

If you have developed a serious problem with alcohol, there are several good organizations that can provide you the help you need. But if your alcohol use does not require this type of assistance, simply bite the bullet and eliminate it completely, at least for the time being.

Using Drugs to Escape

Although alcohol is typically the Avoider's drug of choice, there are many other substances, both legal and illegal, that are frequently used by people with this eating profile.

The abuse of psychoactive prescription medications in this country is no small matter. Millions of people take higher doses of perscription drugs, or use these drugs more often than is prescribed, or use them to "get high" and escape their problems. Nonprescription drugs, including those readily available in drugstores, as well as those illicitly available on the street, also are a target for abuse.

If you have a problem with prescription, nonprescription, or illegal drugs, you must stop abusing these substances, both for your health in general, and to learn the skills you need to overcome your eating problem. If you need professional assistance, get it. If you don't, "just say no" and discontinue their use.

Low Blood Sugar and Problem Solving

When you don't eat on a regular basis, the sugar level in your blood sharply declines. Many people experience difficulty thinking straight and making decisions when their blood-sugar levels are low.

Since you are trying to master the ability to face and solve your problems, it is important that you do not compound your situation by allowing your physical state to work against you. Eat regularly to avoid dips in your blood sugar and you will avoid the pitfalls that hypoglycemic reactions bring.

AFTER COMPLETING THE PROGRAM

As an Avoider, you have a long history of running away from your feelings and avoiding your problems. Overeating has served as your "avoidance strategy," providing you with a way to escape dealing with life's difficulties.

Through this program you have learned new ways of handling your problems. Although you are off to an excellent start, you will need to continue to practice and utilize these newly found abilities. In fact, they need to become lifelong skills.

I personally have a long history of using substances, including, of course, food, to avoid facing problems. In fact, to be honest, it really wasn't until I gave up my final crutch—cigarettes—a number of years ago that I truly can say I developed an ability to confront and solve my problems.

What a different life this has given me! I no longer look toward food, or any other substance, to hide from my problems. Now I acknowledge my feelings and face my problems squarely, with well-thought-out and assertively executed solutions.

Through identifying your problems and then developing and putting forth their solutions you will find that many things change in your life. First, of course, is your weight. You no longer will have the urge to engage in unnecessary eating and overeating, because you now have better, healthier ways of coping with life. Overeating will no longer serve its old purpose, that is, helping you to avoid dealing with life.

By developing this alternative way of approaching everyday difficulties you also will be giving yourself another gift in addition to permanent weight control. You will be giving yourself the gift of self-esteem and self-confidence, which will assist you immensely in almost everything you do. Feeling good about yourself and your abilities is a great feeling—one you are entitled to and deserve!

6

The Energizer: Recharging Your Life

Carla has trouble with her mood. She feels down and tired a lot of the time, even though things are going pretty well in her life. She has a great job, two terrific kids, and a husband who adores her.

But depression runs in her family, so she assumes her mood problem is due to heredity. In addition to depression, she has battled her weight problem for many years.

"When you feel depressed, what to do you do to try to feel better?" I asked her.

"I usually go to the supermarket and buy food I really love. Then I go home and pig out."

Of all the different reasons that people overeat, mood is one of the most common. Like Carla, most people have times when they use food to try to make themselves feel better.

People like Carla, however, do not behave this way just on occasion. They frequently feel depressed and habitually try to lift their spirits with food. While this may help for a little while, in the end they feel even worse than before. Feeling guilty and bad about overeating, they wind up even more depressed.

Feeling "down" is only one symptom of a mood problem. Chronic fatigue (despite adequate sleep) and frequent boredom also are common signs of depression.

If you find that you often are feeling sad, tired, or bored, and you respond to these feelings by eating, it is very likely that you are an Energizer, using food to improve your mood.

Margie, an Energizer I worked with about ten years ago, felt depressed and tired much of the time. Despite the fact that she was an attractive and bright young woman, she perceived herself as unattractive and unintelligent.

Her distorted self-perception could be traced back to her childhood. Margie was raised by an aunt and an uncle in a verbally and physically abusive environment. At thirty-five she continued to carry the self-view that she was ugly and stupid.

When I first met Margie, she was in a job that did not measure up to her abilities, in a relationship with a man who cheated and lied to her, and on probation with a suspended driver's license for a third D.U.I. (Driving Under the Influence). In addition, she was twenty-five pounds overweight, relying on food to raise her mood and energy level on her "down days."

Margie was able, during the course of our six months together, to conquer her mood problem once and for all. She obtained a new job that was much more challenging (and paid considerably more), dumped the loser boyfriend, quit drinking, *and* lost those twenty-five pounds. She lost the weight because she had stopped using food as an antidepressant. She no longer needed to eat to make herself happy, she was able to do that on her own.

Although Margie initially was clinically depressed, not all Energizers have such severe problems with their mood. More minor or subtle mood problems also lead people to overeat.

Regardless of how a mood problem is expressed (sadness, boredom, or fatigue), and irrespective of the severity of the problem, all Energizers must deal directly with their mood if they want to obtain permanent weight control. This is exactly what the psychological approach to overeating accomplishes.

But before we get to the specifics of the treatment program, let's examine some of the factors that contribute to the development of mood problems.

THE CAUSES OF MOOD PROBLEMS

As is the case for most psychological problems, mood problems have both hereditary and environmental factors contributing to their development.

Both clinical depression ("major depression") and more minor forms of depression have a genetic component. While it is clear that individuals born into families with high rates of depression are at increased risk for developing the disorder, exactly *what* is inherited is not clear.

Many researchers have focused on brain neurochemistry as a likely hereditary factor in the etiology of depression. However, while research has shown a strong link between brain chemistry and depression, we do not know whether the neurotransmitter imbalances observed are *cause* or *consequence* of the disorder. In other words, do neurochemical imbalances in the brain cause depression, or are they a consequence or result of having depression?

The focus on neurochemistry and depression has led to tremendous advances in the pharmacological treatment of the condition. The relatively recent development of the specific serotonergic-reuptake inhibitor drugs (SSRIs), the most famous of which is Prozac, has provided relief from depression for many who previously had not responded to treatment.

Other nonpharmacological approaches to treating depression have also been successful, in many cases achieving improvement levels comparable with those obtained with medication.

In particular, cognitive therapies aimed at changing the ways in which people think about themselves and the world have been shown to be highly effective in treating mild to moderate levels of depression. Other forms of psychological treatment, including behavior therapy, interpersonal therapy, and family therapy, also have been shown to work, either alone, or in combination with medication.

Getting back to the causes of mood problems, environmental factors also play a powerful role in the development of depression. For example, research studies have repeatedly found that people who work and who are married are less likely to experience depression than their unemployed and single counterparts. (Of course, being employed and in a relationship certainly is not a guarantee against experiencing depression—people with dissatisfying jobs and bad relationships are usually not very happy.)

Loss experiences, such as losing a significant other through separation, divorce, or death, often precipitate the onset of a mood problem. Perceived failure experiences, such as losing a job, can contribute to developing depression as well.

In addition to our experiences as adults, negative or traumatic events experienced during childhood and adolescence can continue to follow us into our adult lives. Verbal, physical, and sexual abuse, as well as parental physical and emotional neglect, lead to the development of a negative self-image that can be very difficult to shake. Sometimes even extraordinary successes in adulthood cannot counteract chronic feelings of inadequacy that stem from childhood.

Regardless of the reasons why you are experiencing a mood problem, there are many things you can do to turn your mood, and your eating, around. Let's turn to them now.

THE PSYCHOLOGICAL APPROACH
TO DEPRESSION-RELATED OVEREATING

If you are an Energizer, I can promise you this: *Eating will not solve your mood problem.* Although you might feel better briefly (perhaps while you are eating, and for a few minutes afterward), in the end you will feel even worse than before. That is because overeating further fuels your self-dislike. This pattern is very much a vicious cycle: feeling down, eating to feel better, feeling worse because you have eaten, then eating once again because you are feeling bad, and so on.

To become thin and stay thin Energizers must conquer the true source of their overeating—their mood problems. When you develop psychological skills that improve mood, depression-related overeating is eliminated because the negative emotion that triggers this behavior disappears.

The Program for the Energizer includes the specific treatment procedures that will help you conquer your mood problem. The list contains four techniques: two that focus on changing your thoughts, and two that focus on changing your behavior.

In order to change problematic thoughts and attitudes that are characteristic of Energizers, you will learn how to *challenge unhelpful beliefs* and to substitute *positive self-appraisals* for negative self-appraisals. You also will learn how to change your behavior so that you experience more satisfaction in your life, by increasing *pleasurable activities* and setting (and then reaching) *personal goals*.

Program for the Energizer

Treatment Method	Begin
Challenging beliefs	Week 1
Positive self-appraisals	Week 2
Pleasurable activities	Week 3
Personal goals	Week 4

Like the program charts included for the other eating profiles, this chart suggests a timetable to learn the techniques. It is best to learn one treatment method at a time, moving on to the next only after you have become comfortable with the current one.

By mastering these four skills you will gain control of your mood problem. As the symptoms of depression fade, so will your over-involvement with food. You will no longer use eating to counter sadness, boredom, or fatigue. Moreover, your weight loss will be *permanent,* because you will have eliminated the underlying cause of your weight problem once and for all.

LETTING GO OF UNHELPFUL BELIEFS

Through life experiences we develop attitudes and ways of looking at things that guide us through our day-to-day living. These beliefs evolve, to a large extent, as a function of our early experiences, influenced by parents, teachers, and our religious upbringing.

Beliefs can be thought of as helpful or not helpful. Helpful beliefs are those that assist us in conducting our lives in a way that keeps us physically and mentally safe and well adjusted. Unhelpful beliefs, on the other hand, are destructive to our well-being: They cause us to be overly critical and demanding of ourselves, jeopardizing our happiness.

Whether beliefs are helpful or unhelpful can change during the course of our lives. Although a particular belief may have served us well at one point, at a different time in our lives it may no longer function this way.

For instance, a young child living in an abusive environment may learn that keeping quiet and out of the way is the best way to avoid physical harm. However, this type of passive and unassertive behavior will most likely not be helpful to this child when he grows up. As an adult, he will need to change his orientation toward other people, or he will feel helpless and depressed.

Typically people with a tendency toward depression have many beliefs that are unhelpful. Their emotional problems can stem, at least in part, from the unreasonable demands they place on themselves because of their unhelpful beliefs.

Unhelpful beliefs often are unrealistic. For example, beliefs such as "Everyone should like me," or "I should be good at everything," inevitably lead to discouragement and depression because, realistically, they are unobtainable. By maintaining these beliefs, we do ourselves a tremendous disservice, because we will always come up short.

Unrealistic beliefs often include words like *always, never, all,* and *completely.* This type of black-and-white thinking is highly characteristic of people with mood problems.

By contrast, helpful beliefs are realistic. They promote ideas and attitudes that are sensible and produce positive consequences. They tend to be flexible, allowing room for exceptions and special circumstances. Flexible beliefs include multiple gradations of gray, as well as areas for black and white.

Identifying Unhelpful Beliefs

Before you can work on changing your unhelpful beliefs, you need to identify them. Below is a list of beliefs that are common to people with mood problems. Complete the Beliefs Questionnaire and see which ones apply to you.

In addition to absolute terms like *always* and *never,* unhelpful beliefs also frequently include the word *should.* You can discover other unhelpful beliefs that you have by running a mental check on the relationship, events, and activities in your life, and noting which have *shoulds* attached to them.

Are there any *shoulds* attached to the important relationships in your life? Your relationship with your significant other (e.g., "I should always feel in love with my husband"; "I should never argue

---

Beliefs Questionnaire

	Agree	Disagree
1. I should be perfect.	_____	_____
2. I should never make a mistake.	_____	_____
3. Everyone should like me.	_____	_____
4. I should never feel bad.	_____	_____
5. I should put others first.	_____	_____
6. I should be good at everything.	_____	_____
7. I should be nice to everyone.	_____	_____
8. I should always be in control.	_____	_____

---

with my spouse"), children (e.g., "My children should always come first"; "I should be the perfect parent"), family, or friends? How about your work, in or outside of the home (e.g., "I should always enjoy my work"; "My home should always be immaculate")? Do you hold any *shoulds* regarding yourself, including your appearance (e.g., "I should always look good"), personal habits (e.g., "I should never miss a day of exercise"), hobbies, and mental or physical health (e.g., "I should always feel good"; "I should never feel down or upset")?

Identifying your *shoulds* is the first step. The next step is to thoroughly examine each belief and determine whether you think it is unhelpful. It is one thing for me to tell you that a particular belief is unhelpful. It is an entirely different matter for you to acknowledge that the way you have been looking at something does not work and needs to change.

In trying to determine whether a particular belief or attitude is unhelpful, you might want to make a list of the positive and negative consequences that are produced by adhering to the belief. As an example of how to do this, let's take a look at Judy.

Judy is a perfectionist. Perhaps because she was raised by an extremely critical mother, Judy has spent most of her life trying to be the best at everything she does. She learned early on that avoiding mistakes was a way to avoid criticism.

In pursuing perfection, Judy spends hours in front of the mirror, trying to get her hair and makeup just right. In decorating her home, she devotes weeks and months to making selections, to make sure that she is making the perfect choice. At her job, she checks and rechecks her work to be certain that it contains no mistakes.

Despite all the time Judy devotes to her pursuit of perfection, she is never satisfied. Nothing she does ever meets her extremely high standards. As a result, she is depressed a lot of time.

Judy's belief that she must be perfect is not working for her. Rather than enhancing her life, it is ruining her chances for happiness. Not only is she not able to meet this goal, the excessive amount of time she is spending on it is taking away from other things in life that *could* bring her satisfaction.

Changing Unhelpful Beliefs

Once you decide which beliefs are unhelpful and in need of change, the next step is to learn how to challenge them. One way to do this is to come up with "counterarguments" that refute the ideas contained in the unhelpful belief.

For instance, in Judy's case, she might oppose the idea "I should be perfect" with the counterargument: "There is no such thing as perfect. Since perfection does not exist I am spending my time trying to obtain the impossible." Or she might say to herself: "I developed this belief as a child in order to try to protect myself from my mother's criticisms. While it might have been helpful at that time, as an adult my perfectionism is causing me misery."

In developing your counterarguments, it is helpful to write them out. On a piece of paper, list your unhelpful beliefs on the left, and then, directly opposite, on the right, list the counterarguments that you will use to challenge each one.

Whether you recall your counterarguments by memory or refer to this sheet, you need to use them each and every time you encounter your unhelpful beliefs. It will take some practice, but by repeatedly challenging your unhelpful beliefs you will change them.

Remember, as an Energizer, it is your mood problem that is responsible for your overeating. Challenging and eliminating unhelpful beliefs is critical to getting your mood under control, and, consequently, losing the weight, once and for all.

CHANGING NEGATIVE SELF-APPRAISALS

In addition to unhelpful beliefs, Energizers have another way in which they undermine themselves with their thoughts—with negative self-statements, particularly negative self-appraisals.

Self-appraisals—both positive and negative—consist of specific things that we say to ourselves in our heads, our self-statements. Self-statements are somewhat different from beliefs. As discussed in chapter 4, while Stress Reducers tend to have self-statements about danger, the self-statements of Energizers usually take the form of negative self-appraisals.

Negative self-appraisals are the things you say to yourself to put yourself down. Thoughts that start out "I can't," "I'm not," "I won't be able to" usually end up being negative self-appraisals. They are a reflection of low self-esteem and serve to maintain a negative self-view.

By criticizing yourself through your negative self-appraisals you lower your mood and increase the likelihood that you will reach for food for solace.

In order to break this vicious cycle, you need to get out of the habit of putting yourself down and develop a new habit of raising yourself up. You need to change "I can't" to "I can," "I'm not" to "I am," and "I won't" to "I will." In other words, you need to learn to speak nicely to yourself (in your head), acting as though you like and believe in yourself, even if (at this time) you don't.

How do you do that? Well, the first step is to catch your negative self-statements, to notice when you are putting yourself down in your thoughts. This can be difficult, as most of us are not used to paying attention to the fleeting thoughts that go through our minds. (If you also put yourself down out loud, you should work on changing what you say about yourself to other people, as well.)

Some people can get a pretty good idea of the types of negative thoughts they have by making a conscious effort to pay attention to them for a week or two. Most people, however, find that they need to jot down these thoughts as they are happening in order to get hold of them. Use the Negative Self-Appraisal form on the next page to do this. Write down your negative self-appraisals as they happen. In addition, you should supply details, such as where you were when you had the thought, to see if there are any particular situations that commonly trigger these negative thoughts. It may turn out that most of your negative self-appraisals occur in the presence of a particular person or while you are doing a certain activity.

			Negative Self-Appraisal		
Date	**Time**	**Location**	**Activity**		**Negative Self-Appraisals**

Once you have identified your negative self-appraisals you can then work on developing positive self-appraisals that counter the ideas expressed in your negative thoughts. For example, if you think, "I'm not pretty," you might focus instead on some aspect of your physical appearance that you like, such as your hair or your eyes. If you think, "My thighs are fat," you might concentrate instead on your small waist or firm derriere.

In other words, you need to begin to selectively focus on positive aspects of yourself through your self-statements. By doing this, repeatedly over time, the proverbial glass half empty will turn into the glass half full.

On the form opposite, list the positive self-appraisals that you will use to counter your negative self-appraisals. Remember, your positive self-statements will be used to replace your negative self-statements, so the two need to be thematically related.

Developing Positive Self-Appraisals

Negative Self-Appraisals	Alternative Positive Self-Appraisals
Example:	
"I'm not pretty"	"My hair is pretty"
1. _____	1. _____
2. _____	2. _____
3. _____	3. _____
4. _____	4. _____
5. _____	5. _____

Some people have trouble with the idea of refuting negative self-appraisals that they perceive as accurate, for instance, being overweight. However, even if your negative self-statement is true, repeatedly saying it to yourself in your head will not serve any constructive purpose. Saying negative things to yourself makes you feel bad, which leads you to overeat, and, ultimately, to feel even worse than before.

If there are some negative aspects of yourself that you wish to change, these can be tackled by working on personal goals, which we will get to later on in this chapter. Repeatedly criticizing yourself will not help you to change; it only will lead to despair and unhappiness. (Also, if you found, through filling out your record, that certain people, situations, or activities tend to coincide with your negative self-appraisals, this should be addressed in developing your personal goals.)

Learning to replace negative self-appraisals with positive self-appraisals requires practice and persistence. You didn't develop this style of thinking overnight, and it will not disappear suddenly.

Positive self-appraisals are a way of taking care of yourself and expressing self-love. Just as you do certain things to take care of your physical health—brushing your teeth, taking vitamins, getting regular medical checkups—you need to develop a similar conscientiousness about your mental health. Being kind to yourself, through your self-talk, is one way to do this.

ADDING PLEASURE TO YOUR LIFE

One of the things that keeps us going in our daily lives is the reward we get from interacting with people and participating in enjoyable activities and events.

Unfortunately, when people are feeling down they tend to decrease their interactions and activities, withdrawing, to some extent, from the world around them. By decreasing their involvement with their environment, they reduce the pleasure and rewards they receive, and, as a result, can become even more depressed.

Happy, energetic, fulfilled people are active in their environments, obtaining pleasure from the world around them. They incorporate, whenever possible, pleasurable activities into their daily lives, rather than waiting for a special occasion to reward themselves. They value themselves as worthwhile human beings who *deserve* to feel good.

One way in which people obtain pleasure and feel good about themselves is through socializing with other people. Whether it is talking on the telephone, having lunch with coworkers, or stopping by a neighbor's home for a cup of coffee, as human beings we need the company of others, benefiting greatly from these small, everyday interactions.

People who have a tendency toward depression often do not include enough social contact in their daily lives. There are a number of reasons for this. First, individuals with mood problems usually suffer from low self-esteem and, as a consequence, think other people will not like them. In order to avoid potential criticism and rejection, they limit their contact with other people.

Another reason that some Energizers do not socialize enough is because they feel lethargic. You will recall that fatigue is a common symptom of depression, one that can seriously interfere with activity level.

In addition, some Energizers feel that social activities are not "worth the effort," that is, they anticipate they will not experience pleasure from engaging in the activity. This type of negative, pessimistic outlook is highly characteristic of depression-prone individuals.

Jane, a thirty-three-year-old divorced accountant, avoided social activities for all of these reasons. During the work week, she would eat her lunch in her office alone, rather than going out with her office mates. She rationalized her behavior by saying that she thought it best not go get too involved with people she worked with. In reality, however, Jane was afraid that her coworkers would not like her if they really got to know her.

After work and on the weekends, Jane would complain that she was too tired to participate in the social events available to singles in her community. She felt that these activities would be a waste of time, anyway, since it was unlikely she would meet "anyone decent" there.

Jane's minimal social contact was both a cause and a consequence of her depression. She avoided being with other people because of her low self-esteem, fatigue, and pessimism. Unfortunately, by shying away from social activities, she limited the amount of pleasure she received, and continued to be depressed. As an Energizer, this translated into food binges.

In order to get a better idea of the extent to which you include pleasurable social activities into your daily life, keep a detailed record of them for at least a week, using the Daily Social Activities form on the next page.

Complete the record for at least seven days, then take a look at the information it contains. Does it seem that there are certain times or days of the week that you neglect to spend time with other people? Do you limit your social contacts to the telephone, Internet, or other "safe" indirect types of contact? Are your social interactions limited to one or a few select people? Do certain types of social activities consistently produce higher pleasure ratings?

Based on your analysis of the information you recorded, you now should be able to determine how you can best increase your pleasurable social contact. For instance, you may find that you feel terrific every time you talk on the telephone with your long-distance friend Sue. Unfortunately, though, you usually only speak to her on weekends, because of your schedules and the cost of long-distance calls. But maybe the two of your can squeeze in an additional quick call during the week, say at 11:00 P.M., right before bedtime, when the telephone rates go down and you both have a few free minutes.

As another example, your record might reveal that you really enjoy spending time with the other mothers who accompany their children to the weekly "Mommy and Me" class. Why not create another time during the week when all of you (either with or without the children) can get together? Perhaps you can take turns at each others' homes, setting aside one morning each week for an informal get-together.

| | | | Pleasure Rating |
| | | Duration | (0–8; 0 = none, |
Date	Activity	(minutes)	8 = most)

Daily Social Activities

But what if you find that you really don't have much to record on your form, that your daily life pretty much excludes socializing with others? If this is the case, then now is the time to begin adding social activities into your life, spending time with different people and trying out various types of social events.

Is there a local health club or aerobics studio where you might get involved in taking classes and meeting new people? Is there a coworker at the office you could ask out to lunch and get to know better? Is there an old friendship that you have neglected that could be rekindled? Is there a support group in your community where you might get together with other individuals who are faced with similar challenges (depression, single parenting, surviving illness, etc.)?

There are lots of other pleasurable activities in addition to spending time with others. The pursuit of hobbies and special interests, and even involvement with work, can bring great satisfaction and joy. A job well done, whether it is completing an adult education course, playing tennis, or performing volunteer work at a local hospital, increases our sense of competence and self-value.

Tom, a thirty-nine-year-old graphic artist, found that as his career progressed, he spent less and less time on his hobbies and interests. His days were becoming more and more the same, and he complained that he was bored and felt unenthusiastic a lot of the time. He was overeating on a regular basis, trying to alleviate his boredom with food.

Tom recalled that years ago he used to participate in several sports—basketball, tennis, and golf. Being physically active was very enjoyable for him; it provided him with time "with the boys," released tension, and gave him a feeling of accomplishment. Tom also used to spend a good bit of time on his hobby, photography, but somehow that had slipped away as well.

When Tom started reintroducing his hobbies and interests into his life, he experienced a dramatic shift in mood. No longer bored, he was full of energy and enthusiasm. Tom was once again doing the things he loved and was feeling great as a result. His overeating, which had been induced by boredom, stopped, and he returned to his ideal weight.

Are there things that you used to like to do but find you aren't doing anymore? When you were younger, and your life was less hectic, what kinds of hobbies and interests brought you pleasure? Can you, like Tom, reintroduce some of them into your life?

Alternatively, perhaps you have not yet fully explored your potential interests. Many people get so wrapped up in their daily activities—work, maintaining the home, running errands, taking care of the children—that they don't even have time to think about what might be of interest to them. If you are an Energizer, it is very important that you begin to pay more attention to your own personal happiness by expanding your life with hobbies and interests.

Some Energizers I have worked with maintain that they have no hobbies because nothing is particularly interesting to them. Further exploration, however, usually shows that these people have not tried out different activities to see what might be fun for them. Sometimes we don't know that we like something until we actually try it.

If you are one of these people, someone who has trouble identifying what is fun, you need to consider "testing the water" by trying out different types of activities. Take a few golf lessons, sign up for a watercolor class, learn to use a computer. In other words, take a chance and you just might happen upon something new that will add pleasure and interest to your life.

Our personal, private time also can generate pleasure. Reading a good book, taking a hot bath, going for a drive or long walk, all of these are small but meaningful treats that we can give ourselves to increase our daily "pleasure quotient." I like to refer to activities like these as personal pampering. It is one of the best ways to show yourself that you care about yourself.

Even if your life is incredibly hectic, you should be able to find at least a few minutes each day to do something special for yourself. If you find you are resistant to this idea, chances are that your reluctance is due to low self-esteem. Since doing something nice for yourself implies that *you are worth it,* this behavior will conflict with your negative self-view.

To make lasting changes in your self-view you must act "as if," even though you may not really believe it at first. In other words, if you treat yourself "as if" you are worth it, eventually you will come to see yourself in a much more positive light.

The Personal Pampering List will get you to think about small things you can do for yourself each day to feel good. List at least five activities that you can use, as well as the amount of time each takes to complete. (Knowing how long each activity takes helps you to plan where you will incorporate these events into your daily life.) For obvious reasons, do not include eating as a personal pampering activity.

Increasing pleasurable activities—whether social, work, or hobby related, or time alone for pampering—will decrease depression, and, as a result, the overeating that it causes. If you are an Energizer, you must incorporate pleasurable activities into your daily life, even if you literally need to schedule them into each day with the help of a daily planner or calendar.

Personal Pampering List	
Pampering Activity	**Duration**
Example:	
Bubble bath	15–20 minutes
1. _____	_____
2. _____	_____
3. _____	_____
4. _____	_____
5. _____	_____

It's important to remember that the goal here is to increase pleasurable interactions and activities, not ones *you think* you should be involved with but actually do not enjoy (for example, spending more time with a relative you don't really like, or learning to do something you think is important but don't want to do). Those types of activities will be addressed when we get to working on personal goals.

It's also important to recognize that what is pleasurable for you is highly individualized. For instance, you may really love to window-shop at the mall. However, while this activity is extremely enjoyable for you, your spouse may consider it pure torture. On the other hand, your spouse may be totally addicted to playing golf. You, however, consider the game to be incredibly boring.

In summary, there are no right or wrong choices when it comes to increasing pleasurable activities in your life. Interactions and events that make you feel good (that, of course, are not harmful) will counter depression and the overeating it triggers.

PERSONAL GOALS

Are you the person that you want to be? Are there aspects of yourself or areas of your life that could stand improvement?

Almost all of us could easily answer no to the first question and yes to the second. I don't think there is a person alive who doesn't feel he or she could benefit by making changes in some aspect of his or her life.

Although it is normal to see areas in ourselves that could benefit from change, Energizers tend to be especially hard on themselves. Many of their self-criticisms are unwarranted, reflecting thoughts and attitudes that need to be modified, rather than behaviors that need to be changed. The tricky part is distinguishing between the two. Negative self-appraisal is unhelpful and contributes to a depressed mood, while constructive self-criticism can lead to positive change.

Unhelpful beliefs and negative self-appraisals were addressed earlier in this chapter. These are the things that you say to yourself that are unproductive (and usually untrue); only serve to make you feel bad about yourself.

Personal goals, on the other hand, are genuine aspects of your personality or daily living style that can and should, in your opinion, be changed. By making these changes your level of happiness will increase, and you will live a more satisfying life.

Setting and then reaching realistic goals gives us a sense of competence and control over our world. By and large, Energizers tend to be reluctant to set goals for themselves, or if they do, the goals are so unrealistic that they form a foundation for self-recrimination. Fear of failing inhibits them from trying in the first place. This type of avoidant behavior further strengthens the Energizer's view of himself or herself as incompetent or unworthy.

Coming up with personal goals is not a license for self-abuse. The idea here is not to come up with a long list of what is "wrong" with you, but rather to create a few realistic, healthy goals that will add joy or meaning to your life.

How do you decide which goals to pursue? The areas that many people find helpful to focus on include: relationships with others, work (outside or inside of the home), and personal pursuits, including hobbies, habits (e.g., quitting smoking, regularly exercising, reorganizing one's wardrobe, etc.), and skill building (e.g., learning to be more assertive, learning to use the Internet, etc.).

Looking at your relationships first, are you satisfied with your marriage (or relationship with your significant other)? If you do not have a significant other, are there avenues you could be exploring to find that special someone? How about your friendships? Are there acquaintances in your life whom you would like to turn into friends? Are you pleased with the quality of your relationships with other family members, or your children?

If you are employed, are you satisfied with your job? Is there something you could be doing to enhance your job skills and marketability? If you do not work outside the home, would you like to? If you have been working for many years, do you want to be planning for retirement? Are you pleased with the way you are handling your finances and savings?

As for personal pursuits, are there hobbies or interests that you would like to take up? Any bad habits that you want to work on changing (besides overeating)? Any new healthy habits that you want to incorporate into your life? Something new that you want to learn, just for the challenge of it?

Take out a piece of paper and list five personal goals you would like to pursue.

Personal goals can range from relatively small accomplishments, such as deciding to begin taking vitamins on a daily basis, to very large ones, such as going back to school to obtain a degree. Regardless of the size of the goal, in order to succeed it is best to break it down into small parts.

Remember how when you were in school you were taught to make an outline before writing a report? That was good advice, and not only for report writing. Any goal you undertake will be easier and more likely to be completed if you break it down into steps.

For example, in writing this book, not only was the volume broken down into chapters, but each chapter then was divided into multiple sections. Working on the book involved submerging myself in one section of a chapter at a time, not thinking about the whole chapter (or the whole book). In this way a potentially overwhelming task (and believe me, writing a book can be an overwhelming task) becomes a manageable one.

Choose one of the five goals you listed on your paper and break it down into several steps, using the form on the next page. Note that more complex goals usually require more steps.

Obtaining Your Goal

Steps:

1. _____

2. _____

3. _____

4. _____

5. _____

As you accomplish each step of your goal, it is important to reward yourself for completing that part. Remember, reinforcement is a powerful tool that you can use to keep up your motivation level. Just make sure *never* to use food as a reward!

By getting into a new pattern of setting and reaching personal goals your self-esteem will increase. You will have fewer and fewer down times and, as a result, fewer triggers for overeating. Since Energizers overeat when they feel bad, the best defense is to feel good! This is exactly what achieving goals accomplishes.

OTHER THINGS YOU SHOULD KNOW ABOUT

Caffeine and Tobacco

Energizers love their stimulants! As you know by now, both caffeine and nicotine are stimulant drugs that increase autonomic nervous system activity. They increase your heart rate and blood pressure, giving you that surge of "adrenaline" you think you need to get up and going.

Unfortunately, to be very honest with you, it is often quite difficult for Energizers to give up caffeine or cigarettes because of their stimulant properties.

Of course, both are health hazards. What's more, by relying on these substances to pick you up, your likelihood of learning psychological methods for controlling your mood is lessened. Why should you spend the time learning these techniques when you can drink three cups of coffee or have a couple of cigarettes and get the mood lift you are after?

By continuing to rely on artificial means to pick yourself up, you will not have the incentive to learn and master the skills you need to truly conquer your depression-related overeating. In order to really overcome your mood problem you must give up these crutches so you can learn how to "walk" on your own.

Some Energizers experience mood problems that would benefit from prescription medication to alleviate depression. For these individuals, antidepressant drugs should be viewed as a necessary treatment; this should not be compared with the use of over-the-counter drugs, such as caffeine and tobacco, that mask the problem rather than solving it.

Many people, particularly those who are overweight, worry that they will gain weight if they quit smoking. While research supports the fact that quitting smoking lowers the metabolic rate (remember, nicotine is a stimulant drug that increases the "pace" of your bodily functions), this can be overcome by increasing your activity level.

The other reason that people sometimes gain weight when they quit smoking is because they substitute one oral habit for another—in other words, they often begin eating more. However, if you are an Energizer and are following this program, this should not be a problem for you. Since your trigger for overeating is your mood, and since you have developed psychological methods for dealing with this problem, eating will no longer be your answer to what ails you.

Alcohol

Alcohol can become quite a problem for some Energizers. Although actually a *depressant* drug (the effect of alcohol on the body is similar to barbiturates and other types of central nervous system depressants), it is often used by people with mood problems as a form of self-medication.

Although alcoholic beverages initially give you a mood lift, the end result is far from positive. By taking this depressant drug, you can end up feeling even worse than before. Moreover, using this substance will interfere with your learning the psychological skills that you need to permanently solve your mood problem and get control of your eating.

If you are an Energizer you must give up alcoholic beverages. In order to truly learn how to be happy, you must rid yourself of the false sense of OK-ness that alcohol temporarily provides. In order to conquer the destructive thoughts and behaviors that keep you down, you need to face what's wrong, not hide from it with alcohol.

If you have a serious problem with alcohol abuse or dependence, there are many good resources available to help you. Alcoholics Anonymous, for one, has literally been a lifesaver for many Energizers who have gotten into trouble with alcohol.

Blood Sugar, Depression, and Overeating

When your blood-sugar level dips, you may feel tired, irritable, or down. This type of reaction is common when the body experiences a blood-sugar low. Unfortunately for Energizers, these are the very types of symptoms that lead to overeating. For this reason, Energizers need to pay very careful attention to keeping their blood-sugar levels stable. This is best done by eating three well-spaced meals a day or, even better yet, four to six smaller meals a day.

PMS and the Energizer

Many women experience symptoms of PMS before their periods. Sometimes these symptoms include fatigue or a depressed mood. If you are an Energizer, and you get tired or depressed before menstruation, you are at great risk of overeating just before your period. Using your new skills will be particularly important at these times.

Carbohydrates and the Serotonin Connection

Recently, there has been a lot of attention in the media devoted to the relationship between certain types of food and their effects on brain chemistry. Of particular relevance to Energizers is the role of the complex carbohydrates in blocking serotonin reuptake.

Serotonin is a neurotransmitter found in the brain that is related to a sense of well-being. Many of the current, popular antidepressant medications (e.g., Prozac, Zoloft, Paxil) are thought to work by blocking the reuptake (utilization) of serotonin, essentially allowing more of this substance to be available in the brain.

While carbohydrate foods can increase serotonin levels, they also can make you somewhat sedated or sleepy. If you are an Energizer who tends to feel tired a lot of the time, carbohydrates may not be the best food choice for you. Alternatively, if you primarily suffer from a "down" mood, with very little fatigue, you may be able to help elevate your mood by increasing your carbohydrate consumption.

As an aside, the herb St. John's wort has also been purported to alleviate depression by increasing serotonin in the brain. Research conducted in Europe has supported the efficacy of this herb for treating mild forms of depression. However, as of yet, the FDA in this country has not acknowledged the ability of St. John's wort to function in this way. Clinical trials are currently underway here in the United States.

AFTER COMPLETING THE PROGRAM

As an Energizer, you have been using food to alleviate symptoms of a mood problem for a long time. This strategy has not only been ineffective, you have gained weight as a result.

You have learned several new ways to approach your mood problem by changing your thoughts and your behaviors. After about four weeks, you should notice a change in your mood—feeling sad, bored, or tired less often than before. As your mood improves, your eating will decrease. And as you continue to use these techniques, you will find that you keep feeling better and better, and that your overeating will, by and large, disappear.

Getting rid of mood problems is a process. You will need to continue to use the strategies you have learned in this chapter on a regular basis, and not just for a few months, but for always.

This may sound like more than you bargained for. But in actuality, using the self-help procedures in this chapter is pleasurable, not painful. It feels great to be rid of self-defeating and destructive thoughts and beliefs, and to engage in activities that encourage a positive sense of self.

Believe me, I know. Before I got control of my weight, I used to try to make myself happy with food. Whenever I was feeling down in the dumps (which, unfortunately, was fairly often in my younger years), I would treat myself to something tasty. The end result, of course, was that I would then feel even worse than before, because I had "failed" once again. This would provide more fuel for my already low self-esteem, which would lead me to feel down, and to eat once more.

By using the exact same psychological methods that I have outlined for you, I was able to rid myself of my mood problem. In so doing, I no longer used food to pick myself up, because I began to do this on my own. Consequently, the weight came off, and, more importantly, stayed off.

The same will be true for you. The methods that you have learned for combating depression will help you in all facets of your life, not just in controlling your weight. Of course, losing weight, and keeping it off, also will add to your new sense of pride and self-respect. You will become the person that you are entitled to be—thin, happy, and energetic!

7

The Combination Type

Terry was forty-five pounds overweight when I first met him. Initially, he claimed not to know the reasons why he was overeating. After examining the facts, however, it became clear that Terry used food to deal with two different types of negative emotions.

If he felt tense or uptight, Terry ate. Whether he was under a time pressure to get a work assignment done, or trying to break up a fight between his two children at home, feeling stressed invariably led Terry to the refrigerator.

Moreover, feeling sad or down in the dumps led Terry to eat. Unhappy in his job and lonely in his marriage, he regularly used food to try to lift his mood and feel better.

For Terry, both anxious and depressed feelings triggered overeating. He was a combination type overeater.

When you completed and scored the Eating Profile Questionnaire in chapter 1, chances are you found you have more than one of the five eating profiles or, at least, have some of the features of two or more of the profiles.

Like Terry, most overeaters are combination types. They have characteristics of more than one eating profile.

For people with combination eating profiles, different situations trigger different reasons for overeating. While in certain situations overeating is caused by one particular psychological factor, in other situations an entirely different mechanism is at work. In Terry's case, feelings of sadness and tension, experienced at different times, triggered overeating.

Not only might we have more than one psychological factor

leading us to overeat, during different periods of our lives the causes of our overeating can change.

When I first began applying the psychological approach to my own weight problem in the early seventies, the two main causes of my overeating were my eating behavior (fast, impulsive, inattentive eating, characteristic of the Impulse Eater) and using food to reduce tension (the predominant feature of the Stress Reducer).

Although I was successful at tackling these problems back then and keeping them under control over time, a number of years later I found that overeating was sneaking up on me again, but this time for different reasons. I was behaving like the Hedonist (using food for pleasure and entertainment) and the Energizer (using food to lift my mood). As you will see, the Stress Reducer–Impulse Eater and the Energizer–Hedonist are two of the most common combination eating profiles seen in overweight people. Fortunately, applying the psychological techniques for these two eating profiles also was successful.

I have kept my weight under control for over twenty-two years now. In doing this, I have found that I had to remain observant toward my eating, and that I needed to be flexible in my approach. Over the years, I reached for the treatment methods that corresponded to whichever factors were causing me to overeat at that point in time.

To summarize, the reasons you overeat are not static. They can vary across situations and change over time. Therefore, you need to be prepared to utilize different treatment approaches that correspond to all of the factors causing you to overeat at any one time.

PRIMARY AND SECONDARY CAUSES OF OVEREATING

Although most overweight people have more than one cause behind their overeating, not all causes "are created equal."

A cause may be primary or secondary. Primary causes include the main or most pervasive reasons you overeat. Secondary causes, on the other hand, are factors that influence your eating, but not to as great an extent as your primary causes.

Sometimes secondary causes stem directly from primary causes. In these cases, the cause is secondary in terms of its *relationship* to the primary cause, but not necessarily in terms of its degree of *impact* on your eating (as a secondary cause, it can still exert a powerful influence on your eating).

As an example of this, let's look at Alicia. Alicia uses food to pick up her mood when she is feeling down, as is typical of the Energizer. However, she also shows features of the Hedonist—she eats highly caloric foods, slowly and with great relish, to give herself pleasure when she is sad.

Because Alicia's hedonistic eating is selective, that is, she only eats this way when she is depressed, she is not a "pure" Hedonist. Also, because her hedonistic behavior stems directly from her mood problem, it is a secondary cause that results from being an Energizer.

Sometimes the secondary causes of overeating disappear when you treat the primary causes. For example, if Alicia was successful at getting control of her mood problem by using the treatment program for the Energizer in chapter 6, it is possible that her hedonistic eating also might disappear without directly addressing it. Because her pleasure eating stems directly from her mood problem, eliminating the mood problem could simultaneously eliminate the hedonism.

Although there are occasions when you do not have to treat a secondary cause, you often need to tackle both problems separately. That is because treating the primary cause does not always result in changes in a secondary cause—either because the primary cause has not been eliminated completely, or because the secondary cause now has taken on a life of its own, relatively independent of its origin.

(As an aside, this is the same concept as applies to the treatment of coexisting clinical depression and alcohol abuse. In these cases, a depressed person initially uses alcohol to self-medicate, but drinking ultimately becomes a problem in and of itself. At that point, eliminating the original cause of the drinking—the depression—will not be effective. The alcohol problem must be tackled separately.)

COMMON COMBINATION TYPES

If you are a combination type, you will likely need to learn and master techniques from two or more treatment programs. Although this is a lot of work, the payoff most definitely is there. By eliminating all of the factors that cause you to overeat, you will be assured of getting your weight under control for good.

If you need to use more than one treatment program, do not start two (or more) treatment programs at the same time. Undertake one first, and then, when you feel fairly comfortable with the procedures and techniques in that one, move on to the next program. As you embark on a new program, make sure you continue to use and practice all the skills you previously learned, not just the ones you currently are working on.

Which program should you do first? If you have one primary eating profile—a single cause of your overeating that is most pervasive—I recommend you work on the treatment program for that profile before working on programs for secondary profiles. If you have two or more primary profiles, each of which is roughly equal in importance, then begin with the program you feel most motivated or interested in pursuing.

Although theoretically there are of myriad possible combination types (obtained from forming all possible permutations of the five eating profiles), there are four combination profiles that are particularly common among overweight people. These are: the Stress Reducer–Impulse Eater, the Energizer–Hedonist, the Stress Reducer–Energizer, and the Stress Reducer–Avoider.

The Stress Reducer–Impulse Eater shows features of both the Stress Reducer and the Impulse Eater. This combination type eats quickly, impulsively, and inattentively when confronted with stress.

The Energizer–Hedonist displays characteristics of both the Energizer and the Hedonist. This combination type uses high-calorie food to generate pleasure when depressed or bored.

The Stress Reducer–Energizer has characteristics of both the Stress Reducer and the Energizer. This combination type overeats when anxious or depressed.

The Stress Reducer–Avoider behaves like the Stress Reducer and the Avoider. People with this combination profile raise their own anxiety levels by avoiding dealing with their problems, and then try to reduce the tension with food.

Let's take a more detailed look at each of the four most common combination types.

The Stress Reducer–Impulse Eater Combination Type

Raymond is an anxious, impulsive overeater. When he is under stress, he grabs something to eat without thinking, trying to reduce his discomfort with food.

Raymond eats quickly and inattentively, not really enjoying what he's eating. In fact, when he gets this way, it really doesn't matter what he's eating. He's not eating out of hunger or for pleasure. He's trying to get rid of his anxiety and tension, as fast as possible.

Raymond differs from the "pure" Impulse Eater in that he doesn't *always* eat quickly and inattentively. He only acts this way in the face of stress or when he feels tense. Here, being an Impulse Eater is secondary and being a Stress Reducer is primary; the impulsive eating behaviors stem directly from anxiety.

If you are like Raymond and show impulsive and inattentive eating when you are uptight or tense you need to first address your anxiety problem by using the treatment program for the Stress Reducer.

The anxiety-reduction methods in chapter 4 are critical for you to learn ways other than eating to handle stress and decrease your tension. The program will teach you how to minimize the effects of stress, which will lessen your anxiety-triggered overeating.

The treatment program for the Stress Reducer, as you may recall, includes techniques that focus on the feelings, thoughts, and behaviors that cause anxiety. Relaxation techniques—deep muscle relaxation and abdominal breathing—will help you reduce the physiological aspects of anxiety. The thought procedures—coping self-statements and thought-stopping—will help you decrease worrying and upsetting thoughts that create anxiety. Finally, the exposure exercises will show you how to overcome your fears and eliminate the anxiety they trigger.

It is possible that as your anxiety subsides, so too will your impulsive, inattentive eating. Because your impulsive eating only occurs when you are uptight, "curing" your anxiety may do the trick.

Alternatively, this might not be the case. Then you will need to directly tackle your impulsive eating with the treatment techniques for the Impulse Eater. The program will show you how to change your eating behaviors for the better.

The techniques in chapter 2 focus on changing your eating environment and your eating style so that you develop a more attentive, intentional way of eating. By using these procedures, the quick, unthinking eating that appears when you are tense will vanish. Moreover, eating in this new way will help force you to face your anxiety head-on, where you can then practice your antianxiety techniques, rather than turning to food.

Although the anxiety-reduction techniques will help you immensely, there still will be times when major stresses outside of your control occur that do not respond completely to your best efforts. If you are going through a rough period at work, if you are having relationship problems with your family or friends, if someone close to you is going through an illness or other major difficulty, you may find that your anxiety-reduction techniques help you, but do not completely eliminate your tense feelings. It is during stressful times like these that you particularly need to be on the lookout for gobbling, the quick, unthinking grabbing of food that, for you, comes with anxiety.

By using the treatment techniques for the Stress Reducer and the Impulse Eater you will ensure your own success. By conquering both of the causes of your overeating, you will be who you want to be—a thin person, for now and forever!

THE ENERGIZER–HEDONIST COMBINATION TYPE

Laurie has had periods of mild depression for as long as she can remember. Also for as long as she can remember, she has been using food to pick up her mood. Always high in calories, her food treats are carefully planned—she will travel to get them, if necessary, or spend long periods of time preparing them in her kitchen. She eats her special foods very slowly and derives great pleasure from them. Sadly, she has come to rely on these food treats as her main source of pleasure and happiness in life.

People like Laurie have characteristics of both the Energizer and the Hedonist. They use high-calorie foods (high fat and high sugar) as a pleasure source to counter a mood problem. Unlike the "pure" Hedonist, however, this combination type seeks out high-calorie foods only when experiencing feelings of sadness, boredom, or fatigue, the types of feelings that are characteristic of depression. Because hedonistic eating stems from a mood problem, it is secondary to being an Energerizer (the primary problem).

If you turn to high-calorie foods when you are feeling sad, tired, or bored, you probably are an Energizer–Hedonist. You will benefit from first utilizing the treatment program for the Energizer.

Chapter 6 shows you how to get a handle on your mood problem. You will see how you can raise your mood (or increase your energy or interest) by changing your thoughts and your behavior. You will build your self-esteem by eliminating unhelpful beliefs and using positive self-appraisals, and by increasing pleasurable and goal-directed activities.

It is quite possible that as your mood improves you no longer will reach for high-calorie foods. After all, if you no longer feel down, there is no reason to use these foods to try to pick yourself up.

However, it is also possible that your pleasure eating will not entirely disappear as your mood problem improves. If this is the case, you will need to directly address your hedonistic eating by utilizing the treatment program in chapter 3.

The treatment program for the Hedonist teaches you how to use food substitution and portion control techniques to reduce your intake of high-calorie foods. You should apply these methods when you are feeling down (or tired or bored), which are the times when you experience urges for fattening foods.

There is no doubt that the procedures outlined for the Energizer will make a major change in your mood. However, there are always times in life when uncontrollable or unforeseen events occur that bring on periods of sadness (for example, the loss of a loved one). If you are an Energizer–Hedonist, your tendency will be to turn to your "old friends"—your special food treats—for solace. During times like these, pay special attention to the suggestions for the Hedonist so that you don't put on weight. Moreover, giving up your "food crutches" may actually help you face and get past the sad event or situation.

By reducing your mood fluctuations and decreasing your calorie intake when you are depressed, you will get control of your eating and your weight. You will lose the weight and, more importantly, keep it off, because you will have learned new, healthy ways to deal with both of the causes of your overeating.

THE STRESS REDUCER–ENERGIZER
COMBINATION TYPE

Kay eats in the face of anxiety *and* depression. When she is feeling stressed, she eats to relax. When she is feeling down, she eats to try to pick her mood up. Kay is dealing with her uncomfortable, unpleasant feelings with food. She tries to alleviate both of these negative emotions through eating.

In a way, Kay is trying to obtain emotional equilibrium. Food is used to keep her on an even keel—to bring her up when she is down, and to bring her "down" when she is wound up.

Difficulties with tension and sadness commonly appear together much more frequently than would be expected by chance alone. Moreover, overeating is a common way people who suffer from tension and sadness try to help themselves. It is a form of self-medication, not all that different from turning to drugs or alcohol for relief.

If you find that you frequently respond to both anxious and depressed feelings by eating, you probably have this combination type. For the Stress Reducer–Energizer, both eating profiles are primary, exerting relatively equal, but independent, effects on eating.

As a Stress Reducer–Energizer, you must learn how to deal directly and constructively with your anxious and depressed feelings rather than trying to eliminate or suppress them with food. The habit of responding to uncomfortable internal states (other than actual hunger) by eating can be changed through developing the psychological skills contained in chapters 4 (The Stress Reducer) and 6 (The Energizer). Because both problems are primary and unrelated, you will need to use both treatment programs.

Chapter 4 shows you a variety of ways to reduce stress and tension, including relaxation exercises, cognitive (thinking) techniques, and exposure procedures. Chapter 6 helps you build your self-esteem and eliminate your mood problem by changing your thoughts and behavior.

By eliminating the two causes of your overeating—anxiety and depression—you will stop overeating and lose weight. Moreover, you will maintain your weight loss permanently, because you will have gotten to the heart of your eating problem.

THE STRESS REDUCER–AVOIDER
COMBINATION TYPE

Charlotte is a tense person who avoids situations that trigger stress or anxiety. In particular, she avoids facing and dealing with her problems—difficulties with her marriage, her children, her job—by denying their existence. Because she is unassertive and lacks problem-solving skills, the idea of directly handling conflicts and problems causes her intense anxiety. By not facing her problems, she reduces her anxiety, at least for the short run.

Charlotte has characteristics of the Stress Reducer and the Avoider. She is an anxious individual who becomes even more anxious when confronted with a problem. As a result, she avoids facing the problem in order to reduce her anxious feelings. Unfortunately, this approach actually makes matters worse. By not addressing the problem it lingers unsolved, producing even more anxiety. Her response to these feelings is to eat.

Being a Stress Reducer and an Avoider are closely intertwined for Charlotte. She avoids stressful life situations to reduce her tension but, in so doing, actually maintains and sometimes escalates her already high level of anxiety. Although avoiding dealing with her problems has the immediate effect of making her feel better (having escaped dealing with an anxiety-producing situation or event), in the long run her avoidance behavior is actually strengthening her anxiety by reinforcing it.

If you are like Charlotte, then you probably are a Stress Reducer–Avoider. Here, both eating profiles are primary and related, with each influencing the other: Anxiety produces avoidance, and avoidance maintains anxiety. To eliminate overeating, this combination profile must use the treatment plans for both the Stress Reducer and the Avoider.

To permanently overcome your weight problem, you must learn the techniques for decreasing anxiety and tension (chapter 4), and also learn how to effectively confront and solve your problems (chapter 6). Again, it is imperative that both of these two treatments are utilized. Because anxiety leads to avoidance behavior (it causes you to run from your problems), and because avoidance behavior strengthens anxiety (avoiding dealing with your problems causes you to continue to be anxious), your overall level of tension and your ability to confront and solve stressful problem situations must be individually and directly addressed.

Avoidance behavior is a hard strategy to break. Because it seems so effective in the short run, you will be tempted to continue to use it. However, if you really understand how avoiding your problems leads to more anxiety and tension in the long run, it will help motivate you to learn how to confront and solve your problems.

Through learning how to deal with your anxiety, and developing the ability to confront your problems, you will get control of your weight. By eliminating both of the causes of your weight problem, you finally will become the thin self you deserve to be.

Treating Three or More Problem Areas

The four combination types we have covered were included in this chapter because they are the most common combination eating profiles seen among overweight people. However, as I mentioned earlier, there actually are numerous possible combination types, consisting of any two, three, four, or even all five of the eating profiles.

For example, there are many overweight people who meet the criteria for the Stress Reducer, the Energizer, *and* the Avoider. These individuals overeat in response to anxiety and depression, and also use avoidance as a way of not dealing with their problems. Moreover, to further compound the situation, this multiple combination type often shows features of the remaining two eating profiles—the Impulse Eater and the Hedonist. They may display impulsive, inattentive eating (the Impulse Eater) when stressed and pleasure eating (the Hedonist) when depressed. Thus, people who fall into this category exhibit behaviors that touch on all five of the eating profiles, albeit varying in degree.

As I discussed in chapter 1, fortunately, the number of profiles you have is not related to your likelihood of success. Whether you succeed depends almost entirely on your willingness to work on and change behaviors and traits that lead you to overeat, no matter how many or how few there are. To gain permanent control of your weight you must completely and accurately identify and understand all of the factors that contribute to your overeating. Then, by addressing each, using the appropriate psychological techniques, you will be in a position to eliminate them, one by one.

Remember, whether you overeat because of one, two, three, four, or even all five reasons, you have just as good a chance to enjoy lifelong weight control as anyone else. Learn your new skills, practice them religiously, and reap your rewards!

8

The Psychological Benefits of Exercise

Let's face it, most of us hate to exercise. Our reasons may be different—it's too boring, too time consuming, or too much work—but the end result is the same: overweight people living sedentary lives.

Most of the time, discussions of the benefits of exercise focus on the positive physical effects of increasing one's activity level. For overweight people, this primarily is the relationship between energy expenditure and weight loss.

While there is no doubt that exercise can contribute to weight loss by burning calories, I want to give you a different vantage point. I am concerned with the psychological health benefits that exercise produces. This is because it is your mental wellness, or lack thereof, that is related to your eating and your weight.

A substantial amount of research has demonstrated the mental-health advantages of regular exercise. Exercise is effective at reducing your overall level of anxiety and tension, as well as reducing the effects of outside stresses. It raises your energy level and counters mood problems. It can provide peaceful time alone that can be useful for problem solving (jogging, for example), or give you a social outlet to interact with other people (when playing sports, for instance).

Basically, there are two kinds of exercise: aerobic and anaerobic. Aerobic activities include those that accelerate your heart rate into a "target zone" where oxygen is utilized most efficiently. Aerobic exercise stimulates the respiratory and circulatory systems, and produces enzymes involved in the metabolism (burning) of fat. Usually, an activity must produce an elevated heart rate continuously for at least fifteen minutes to be considered aerobic. Some common aerobic activities include jogging, bicycling, jumping rope, swimming, singles tennis, and cross-country skiing.

Aerobic activities often are thought of as the exercises or sports that cause people to sweat and be out of breath. However, low-impact, low-intensity aerobic activities have gained popularity in recent years that are not as rigorous as the original aerobics classes people participated in some years back.

In contrast, anaerobic activities do not utilize oxygen like aerobic activities, and do not produce a consistent high heart rate. They either are less demanding overall, such as taking a slow walk or playing golf, or are performed in short, intense spurts, such as weight lifting or playing doubles tennis.

Most of the research that has been conducted on the mental-health effects of exercise has included aerobic activities. One reason for this is that aerobic activities trigger the release of endorphins that produce an overall feeling of well-being.

However, despite the aerobic-endorphin connection, I believe there are significant positive, psychological effects to both kinds of physical activity. Weight lifting, for example, an anaerobic activity, can increase individuals' perceptions of their own strength, control, and competence. Moreover, it is extremely effective for reducing the muscular tension that often is a reaction to stress.

In general, I do not favor one type of exercise over another. Rather, I believe the key is to *match the type of exercise to the individual,* considering both that person's personality traits and psychological strengths and weaknesses. Your exercise plan needs to be individualized in much the same was as your weight-loss approach, according to your eating profile.

The personality traits of the person suggest which type of activities are most likely to be adhered to for an extended period of time. The psychological strengths and weaknesses of the person indicate which type of activities will produce the greatest psychological benefits for that individual.

In this chapter, I outline the types of physical activities that are best suited to each of the five eating profiles. I encourage you, armed with your new knowledge, to develop your own fitness plan, tailored specifically to you.

THE IMPULSE EATER

Impulse Eaters are high-energy individuals who are frequently on the move. They are easily bored and will not tolerate repetitious, monotonous, slow-moving exercises. The idea of plugging away on a treadmill or stationary bicycle seems "meaningless" and would bore them to tears. Rather, Impulse Eaters respond best to sports, usually ones that are fast paced, competitive, goal directed, and social in nature.

If you are an Impulse Eater you are most likely to benefit from and stick with a sport as a physical activity. Consider a vigorous, one-on-one sport, such as tennis (singles), racquetball, or squash, or a team sport, like basketball. If you are out of shape or older, you might want to pursue an activity that requires less energy, such as doubles tennis, golf, or a sport like volleyball or softball.

Because Impulse Eaters tend to be easily bored, it is also a good idea to mix up your physical activities, say have a tennis game once a week and play golf once a week. Also, vary the people with whom you play.

Greg is an Impulse Eater who is in his mid-sixties. He has been a weekend tennis player for years. Recently, after having a health scare, he purchased a treadmill so that he could exercise every day.

Despite the best of intentions, Greg's treadmill is slowly collecting dust in the corner of his bedroom. This nonsocial, noncompetitive activity was simply too boring for him. To increase his frequency of physical activity, he would have been better off scheduling additional tennis games (or some other sport) during the week.

Pursuing sports is also helpful to the Impulse Eater because sports demand attention and concentration, and, to some extent, self-discipline. These are exactly the behaviors the Impulse Eater needs to apply to eating!

THE HEDONIST

Hedonists are out for pleasure. To get Hedonists to exercise on a regular basis is a difficult task—they will only do it if it feels good.

Most exercise does not feel good (at least in the way the Hedonist interprets such feelings). One notable exception, however, is aerobic activity. If an aerobic activity is pursued long enough—usually about twenty minutes—a sense of well-being is experienced, caused by the release of endorphins (also known as a "runner's high").

The problem here is that many Hedonists will not stick with an aerobic activity long enough to experience a "high." As Hedonists, they are motivated to seek pleasure, but have a hard time delaying gratification. They need more immediate satisfaction, a good feeling that comes early on in the activity or exercise process.

If you are a Hedonist, you most likely will benefit from and stick with activities that appeal to your senses, that is, those that "feel good." If you live in a warm climate, and enjoy the feeling of the sun or the fragrance of flowers in the air, gardening might be for you. If you find the sensation of water on your skin soothing and refreshing, you might want to consider swimming. If you enjoy the scenery of the outdoors, walking or jogging may be for you. Any activity that provides a "sensual delight"—be it sight, smell, feel, or sound— would be a good pick for a Hedonist.

One Hedonist I know who lives in a semitropical environment likes to run on the beach. The roar of the ocean and the feeling of the sun's rays on her skin provide her with pleasure for her senses. Because she enjoys the activity, she pursues it long enough to reach a "runner's high," which gives her an additional reward and future incentive for her efforts.

As a Hedonist, if it feels good you are more likely to do it. The corollary is, of course, if it does not feel good, you are not going to do it. Picking a physical activity that brings pleasure to your senses greatly increases the likelihood that you will make it a part of your daily life plan. Moreover, it will provide you with an alternative way of deriving pleasure, one that is much better for you than overeating.

THE STRESS REDUCER

There is no question that exercise can play a powerful role in reducing the tension and anxiety experienced by the Stress Reducer. Both the feeling and thought aspects of anxiety can be dramatically improved with certain types of physical activities.

If you are a Stress Reducer, aerobic activities are a great way for you to decrease your overall level of tension as well as your physiological response to stressful situations. Aerobic activity decreases your autonomic nervous system activity, lowering your heart and respiration rates.

Any aerobic activity that appeals to you will work. If you are not used to exerting yourself physically, you might consider starting with walking. Begin slowly at first, then pick up the pace as you get more accustomed to exercising. Ultimately, you should end up at a very brisk pace that gives you an aerobic workout.

Weight lifting—with either free weights or machines—is terrific for reducing muscular tension that frequently is experienced by Stress Reducers. By concentrating on the tense feelings in your muscles when you are holding the weight, and then contrasting this feeling to the "loose" or relaxed state of your muscles after you have let the weight go, you can achieve benefits similar to those obtained from deep muscle relaxation (see chapter 4).

Because aerobic exercise and weight lifting are both helpful for reducing the physical signs of anxiety, I recommend doing them well into the day—for example, at lunchtime or before dinner—rather than first thing in the morning. By doing them after the stresses and strains of the day's events have begun to affect you, you will get the maximum antianxiety benefits these activities have to offer.

Another physical activity that is good for Stress Reducers is yoga. The stretching that is part of yoga is great for alleviating muscle tightness due to tension. As importantly, the meditation aspects of yoga are very helpful for clearing the mind of worries and upsetting thoughts, problems that frequently are experienced by Stress Reducers.

Doing all three kinds of activities—aerobic exercises, weight lifting, and yoga classes—may be more than you can fit into your schedule. If this is the case, base your selection of activities on the way that you usually experience anxiety. If you have a lot of autonomic nervous system symptoms of tension—increased heart rate or blood pressure, sweating, feeling jittery, pacing—integrate aerobic exercise into your everyday life. If muscle tension is the main way you react to stress, go with weight lifting. Finally, if you are troubled by worries and upsetting thoughts, yoga will be your best bet.

Some Stress Reducers are perfectionists or very sensitive to failure. If you have either of these traits, you probably should not use sports as a physical activity. Worrying about how well you are doing the activity will defeat the purpose of doing it in the first place: It will stress you out, rather than relax you. Also, if an activity causes you anxiety, you will be likely to discontinue it in time.

THE AVOIDER

Most Avoiders are unassertive and lack self-confidence. For them, physical activities can play an important role in helping develop feelings of competence and self-confidence.

Weight training and the martial arts are very useful for assisting the Avoider to build self-confidence. Both of these activities foster feelings of power and control, increasing the psychological perception of oneself as strong and competent.

In weight training, strength and endurance is developed by repeatedly lifting heavier weights over time. Being able to lift progressively larger amounts of weight, and seeing muscles develop in your body, runs counter to the Avoider's typical self-perception of him- or herself as weak and ineffective.

The mental and physical discipline that are part of many of the martial arts (for example, tae kwon do) are beneficial for many Avoiders. Insecurity and indecisiveness, two traits common among people with this eating profile, are at odds with the types of behaviors expected in these activities. For this reason, the martial arts are terrific confidence boosters.

One of the most dramatic psychological changes I have ever observed as a result of a physical activity was when Ann, a lifelong Avoider, took up karate. In a matter of few months, Ann was transformed from the proverbial "wimp" into "superwoman." As her knowledge and abilities in karate increased, so did her view of her own personal effectiveness.

Avoiders also can benefit from taking on a sport as a physical activity. Developing competence at a sport can build self-confidence, but not if you perceive yourself as doing poorly. If you do decide to pursue a sport, make sure that you have some ability in that area and that you are paired with players who are at your same level. The idea here is for you to feel good about yourself and your abilities, not to provide an opportunity to feel like a failure.

If you are an Avoider, taking on weight or martial arts training, or becoming competent at a sport, can help you develop the confidence you need to face your problems. Try it and see!

THE ENERGIZER

The Energizer can be a difficult individual to get going on a fitness plan. Because Energizers often are tired and lack motivation, they frequently complain that they do not feel up to exercising. Moreover, because they are commonly pessimistic, they are skeptical that exerting themselves by exercising will pay off.

If you are an Energizer, you will be best off starting with a less demanding exercise (such as walking), and then working up to more vigorous activities over time. The goal is to get you into aerobic activities, because they are most effective at increasing endorphins—the mood-enhancing brain chemicals that produce a state of well-being.

As a general rule, Energizers should exercise in the morning, when they are rested and alert. Later on in the day, having completed your daily activities, you are more likely to be tired and therefore less likely to do your exercise.

Start slowly! The biggest obstacle for many Energizers is that they begin by demanding too much of themselves, are subsequently disappointed, and then stop exercising altogether. You are much better off initially setting goals that are *too easy* for you, rather than ones that are too difficult. It is critical that you experience early success with your new fitness program, otherwise you very likely will discontinue it.

Avoid doing exercises or participating in sports where you are likely to perceive yourself as "failing." Because Energizers tend to be self-critical and have low self-esteem, thinking you are bad at something or don't measure up to others will only add to your problems—your mood will go down and your eating will go up.

Aerobic activities increase energy and are mood stabilizers. They are tremendously helpful for people all along the depression spectrum, from those with relatively minor mood problems ("moody"), all the way to those with severe, clinically diagnosed depressions. They help energize people who tend to be sluggish or lethargic, as well as those suffering from extreme forms of enduring fatigue (chronic fatigue syndrome).

Recommended Activities by Eating Profile

Activity	Impulse Eater	Hedonist	Stress Reducer	Avoider	Energizer
Badminton				X	
Bicycling		X	X		X
Calisthenics			X		X
Dancing		X	X		X
Gardening		X			
Golf	X				
Jogging		X	X		X
Jumping rope			X		X
Martial arts				X	
Racquetball	X		X		
Rowing			X		X
Running			X		X
Softball				X	
Stair climbing			X		X

Activity	Impulse Eater	Hedonist	Stress Reducer	Avoider	Energizer
Skiing:					
Water		X			
Downhill	X	X			
Cross country		X	X		X
Swimming		X	X		X
Tennis	X		X		X
Volleyball				X	
Walking		X	X	X	X
Weight lifting			X	X	
Yoga			X	X	

When I first met Amy she was feeling tired and down much of the time. As an Energizer, she was using food to try to feel better, but, of course, only ended up feeling worse, eating too much and gaining weight.

I finally convinced Amy to begin a fitness program, starting with walking slowly for five minutes. Over time, Amy picked up her pace and increased the length of her walks. She began to experience more and more energy, and found that she was less moody than before.

Today, three years later, Amy is an avid runner who participates in local marathons. She looks forward to her morning runs, and attributes them, in large part, with helping her maintain her weight loss—not because of the calories she burns, but because of the positive psychological effects this activity has on her everyday life.

The chart on pages 164–165 indicates the specific types of activities that are best suited to each of the five eating profiles. Look it over carefully and then use the Weekly Activity Plan and Record to develop and keep track of a fitness program for yourself.

At the top of your Weekly Activity Plan and Record, list up to three physical activities that you want to do for a particular week. Then, in the "planned" column, note which activities you plan to do on which days, by placing a check mark in the appropriate spot. To keep track of how well you adhere to your plan, use the "actual" column to record what you have done each day, again using a check mark.

Weekly Activity Plan and Record

Week of:_____

Activities

No. 1: _____

No. 2: _____

No. 3: _____

Day	Planned			Actual		
	No. 1	No. 2	No. 3	No. 1	No. 2	No. 3
Monday						
Tuesday						
Wednesday						
Thursday						
Friday						
Saturday						
Sunday						

ACTIVE LIVING

Being active, whether you are engaged in aerobic or anaerobic activities, whether you are pursuing hobbies, sports, or working out at a health club, is part and parcel of what it means to be alive.

In my opinion, it is almost impossible to experience optimum mental health, and an overall feeling of well-being, if you are a sedentary person.

Inactivity tends to add to anxiety and depression. As you have discovered, these emotions are two of the leading causes of overeating, responsible for the weight problems of millions of Stress Reducers and Energizers.

Moreover, anxiety and depression are the two most common psychological problems that lead adults to seek the services of mental-health professionals. While certainly one cannot expect exercise alone to prevent mental-health problems, one can expect it will decrease their likelihood. (In this respect, it is similar to the relationship between smoking and heart disease. Although quitting smoking will not ensure that you do not develop heart disease, it certainly will decrease your odds.)

Not only is exercise helpful for the mental health of the Stress Reducer and the Energizer, people with the other three eating profiles benefit as well. Pursuing a physical activity increases the self-confidence of the Avoider; it provides an alternative, healthier way for the Hedonist to derive pleasure; and it teaches the Impulse Eater to focus attention and concentrate.

In short, all five of our eating types will reap psychological rewards by living active lives.

9

When the Thin Lady Sings!

Susan can't believe she's actually thin. Having been chubby during childhood, fat during adolescence, and obese as a young woman, she is amazed by the attractive, slender woman who looks back at her from the mirror.

Many things have changed in her life as a result of losing weight. Now she has lots of dates and lots of friends. She is self-confident and takes on challenges, both at and outside of work. She feels energetic and alive, looking forward to each and every day.

Because she has tackled the real causes behind her overeating, Susan knows she will stay thin. Finally, she has gotten to the heart of her problem, eliminating the emotions and behaviors that were standing in her way.

By the time you read this chapter, if you have followed the treatment plan for your eating profile you will have lost weight. For those with a lot of weight to lose, you will have gotten off to a great start, shedding those initial pounds and heading toward your optimum weight. For others, who had less weight to lose, many of you will already have reached your goal.

Losing weight is a very positive experience. It gives you a strong sense of power and control. Moreover, it leads you to believe that since you CAN take control of your eating, you can successfully manage other things in your life as well.

I remember the feelings I experienced when I first lost weight twenty-two years ago. For the first time in my life, I was in charge of what I ate; food was no longer in charge of me. Not too long ago I experienced the same sense of empowerment when I quit smoking. I remember thinking, "If I can do this, I can do anything!"

Giving up something you love, something you have used repeatedly for a long time to deal with life, is a difficult task. Hopefully, the psychological approach contained in this book has made it easier for you. By focusing on the underlying psychological factors that lead you to overeat rather than on your food we have eliminated the fear of potential deprivation that comes with more traditional weight-loss approaches, such as dieting.

Nevertheless, I know it hasn't been easy. Dealing with the psychological issues that cause you to overeat is hard work, and in some ways is more threatening than simply focusing on what you eat. Dealing with psychological issues requires you to look at the thoughts, feelings, and behaviors that are part of who you are.

Despite this, you have had the courage to face and overcome the psychological factors behind your overeating. For this you deserve congratulations and praise.

WHAT TO EXPECT AS A THIN PERSON

There are many great things that happen as a result of losing weight.

As I have already mentioned, losing weight is a tremendous confidence builder, giving you a sense of personal empowerment. Following weight loss, you will experience increased feelings of self-esteem and self-worth. You may feel like you now can do things you couldn't do before—taking on new responsibilities and challenges at work, increasing your social activities, and developing new hobbies and interests. If you have other "addictive-type" behaviors (smoking, drinking, etc.), you may decide that this is the time to tackle them as well.

You will feel better about your appearance. In the summertime, you no longer will avoid going to the pool or the beach because you are embarrassed to put on a swimsuit. You will enjoy shopping for clothing rather than dreading it (even those horrendous lights and mirrors in the department store fitting rooms won't deter you). You will take an interest in fashion and look forward to dressing up, because now you will look just as good as the slim people you always have admired.

In addition to changing the ways in which you see yourself, other people may react differently toward the new thin you. When people lose weight they often find they elicit more interest from the opposite sex. Either because they think they are more attractive, and act accordingly, or because they actually are more attractive, thin people are noticed more and have more opportunities for dating.

After you lose weight, you may find that more people are "drawn" to you, that you more easily make friends and that more people want to be your friend. You will find yourself comfortable with same-sex friends of any weight, not only those who are overweight.

Overall losing weight increases one's energy level. You will find you are more active than you were before, tire less easily, and, in general, have more zest and pep for life. (Of interest: Some people comment that their sex lives improve after weight loss. This may be because of better feelings about their bodies, or because they have more energy and physical stamina.)

If you were morbidly obese, once you lose the weight you will find that you no longer are discriminated against. People no longer will treat you as a "second-class citizen" or like a freak. They won't stare, point, or whisper about you. People will want to be around you—hire you, date you, and be your friend. You will be able to travel comfortably, fitting into those narrow airplane seats. You will be able to participate in activities that previously were unavailable to you because of your size and lack of physical endurance.

On a final note, losing weight will have a major, positive effect on your physical health. Losing even ten pounds increases one's life expectancy and decreases one's chances of facing medical conditions and illnesses that are common with advanced age.

In short, many good things happen to those who lose weight.

I have summarized many of the positive consequences of weight loss into the following list. You may want to make a photocopy of the list and place it in a location where you can see it often.

Positive Consequences of Losing Weight

1. You feel empowered, as if you can do things you couldn't do before.
2. Because of your increased self-confidence, you take on new responsibilities and challenges at work and in your leisure time.

3. You are more outgoing and increase your involvement in social activities.
4. You feel more attractive. Your new self-view is shared by the opposite sex, who are now more interested in you.
5. If you were obese, new job opportunities open up to you. You are no longer discriminated against because of your weight.
6. You have more energy and physical stamina.
7. You have improved your mental and physical health and increased the probability of a long and happy life.

Before we finish discussing some of the things you can expect when you are thinner, I would like to briefly mention some other types of reactions that sometimes occur. It is quite possible, or even probable, that none of these things will happen to you. However, I think it is worthwhile to inform you about them, so that you can be prepared in advance, in the unlikely event that any of them do occur.

On occasion, some people who lose weight experience negative reactions from those around them. For instance, particularly if you were very overweight, you may find that your friends who are still overweight who have not joined you in doing this program may be uncomfortable around you. When this happens, it usually is because your success makes them feel like a failure in comparison. Looking at you with your new slim body is a reminder that they have not achieved their goals.

Also, it may be possible that your new, thin self has less in common with your overweight friends than you used to. As a thin person, you no longer will focus on eating as a primary activity in your life. Through this program, you will have developed a different way of approaching life, and have new and varied interests that do not include food. Your friends, however, have not experienced these changes; they may still consider going out for milk shakes, fries, and burgers the perfect evening activity.

On the positive side, if you handle it right, this can be your opportunity to do something truly wonderful for your friends. Encourage them to read this book and help them experience the same success you have!

It may be possible that some people—relatives, friends (who really weren't friends), and acquaintances—will be jealous of what you have achieved. They may act aloof toward you or become critical of you (on nonweight issues). Taken to the extreme, they may actively try to sabotage you, by putting roadblocks in your path, hoping you will cave in and gain back the weight.

If any of these things should happen to you, the first thing to do is to recognize where it is coming from. Individuals who respond this way to other people's successes generally are themselves unhappy and dissatisfied people. In this regard, try to show them some compassion. If they are overweight, they, too, may be candidates for this program.

On a final note, sometimes it is not others' attitudes toward you that become a problem but rather your attitude toward others. Occasionally, newly thin individuals take on a holier-than-thou attitude, seeing themselves as "better" than other people, particularly those who have been unsuccessful in their attempts to lose weight.

If you find that you are acting in this way, try to remember that it was not too long ago that you too were out of control with your eating. Try to help others benefit from what you yourself have learned!

By pointing out problems that some people occasionally face when they lose weight, I do not mean to discourage you or minimize your accomplishment. The potential negative consequences that I have discussed are simply possible reactions to a thin you, ones that probably won't occur, but, nevertheless, ones you may want to look out for.

By far, the advantages of losing weight well exceed any potential disadvantages. The mental and physical health benefits alone make it one of the most important changes you probably will ever make in your life.

AVOIDING SETBACKS AND RELAPSES

Hundreds of research studies have shown that losing weight is not nearly as difficult as maintaining weight loss after it has occurred. For traditional weight-loss approaches, i.e., diets and other nutritional plans, when it comes to maintaining weight losses, relapse is the rule rather than the exception.

There is no question that your risk of gaining back the weight is much less than people who lose weight by focusing on food. Unlike traditional weight-loss plans, your treatment program has taught you how to deal effectively with the emotions and behaviors that lead to overeating. By addressing the real, underlying reasons behind your weight problem, rather than the symptom expression of these problems (overeating), you are in a much better position to keep the weight off.

The potential problem for you comes if you discontinue using your treatment techniques. As I have repeatedly pointed out throughout this book, your treatment techniques are intended to be used as lifelong skills, not temporary "fixes."

Granted, eventually some of these skills will become second nature and turn into habits. When this happens you won't need to consciously think about using your skills—you will use them automatically, as the need arises.

There will be some procedures, though, that do not as readily become habits. They require more of your attention for a longer period of time. You will have to make a concerted effort to remember to use them, month after month, year after year.

To help you do this, I encourage you to keep a log detailing the use of your techniques, particularly those that have not yet become habits, with the help of the Self-Monitoring Form on the next page.

At the top of the form, list up to three techniques that you want to keep track of for a particular week. Then indicate whether you used each technique on a particular day of the week by placing a check (did use the technique) or an X (did not use the technique) in the column corresponding to that technique (No. 1, No. 2, No. 3).

Over time, you may find that you become rusty at using a particular technique, either because you have not been faithful in practicing it or because, by happenstance, there have not been that many opportunities to use it. If this happens to you, consider having "booster sessions." Booster sessions simply are appointments that you schedule with yourself to brush up on or relearn a skill.

If you decide to conduct booster sessions, set aside some time and turn to the directions for using that procedure. Approach the skill as if you are learning it for the first time, filling out any questionnaires, completing the forms, and doing assignments. If you really acquired the skill in the first place, you will become comfortable and competent with it much faster the second time around.

Self-Monitoring Form

Week of:_____

Techniques to be monitored:

No. 1: _____

No. 2: _____

No. 3: _____

Day	No. 1	No. 2	No. 3	Notes
Monday _____				
Tuesday _____				
Wednesday _____				
Thursday _____				
Friday _____				
Saturday _____				
Sunday _____				

Another good time to use booster sessions is when you anticipate a potential "threat" to your new way of life—for instance, if you are going on a cruise where you will be tempted by one heavy meal after another. By conducting booster sessions before the trip, your skills will be "fresh" and close at hand, increasing the likelihood that you will use them when faced with temptation. (By the way, many of the major cruise lines offer low-calorie meals as an alternative meal choice. Just have your travel agent place your request sufficiently far in advance.)

You also may find that you can benefit from brushing up on your skills during particularly stressful or difficult times. It is human nature to go back to our old, familiar ways of doing things at such times, particularly if not a lot of time has passed since you completed the treatment program (i.e., your skills are still relatively new).

The only way to avoid setbacks and relapses is to continue to use the psychological tools for your particular eating profile. Self-monitoring and booster sessions are two ways for you to make sure that you keep up your new skills and don't slip back into old patterns. Do not develop a false sense of security in which you think you no longer need to use your skills!

When you reach your weight-loss goal, please remember how you got there—by working hard at changing feelings, thoughts, and behaviors that were standing in your way. Keep on doing this and you will hold on to the new you. I know because I am still there, twenty-two years later.

WHEN THE THIN LADY SINGS

I know that it probably took a tremendous leap of faith and a good deal of courage to try a weight-loss approach that does not focus on food. All of our lives we have been bombarded with diets and weight-loss fads that center on what we eat. Virtually all of them have given us the same message: If you want to lose weight, change what you eat.

Well, we did change what we ate, but still we were not able to lose weight and keep it off. Little did we know that we were not at fault. Rather, the fault lay with the weight-loss approach.

As you have discovered, the vast majority of overeaters are not overweight primarily because of *what* they eat (except the Hedonist). They are overweight because of *how* (their eating began) and *why* (their emotional triggers to eating) they eat. They never will gain control of their eating and their weight with diets or programs that focus on food.

Unlike the millions of dieters across this country, you can conquer the roots of your eating problem. You have seen how to identify the psychological factors that cause you to overeat, and then systematically address each one, using the appropriate psychological self-help techniques specifically designed for them. If you face your problems head-on, you will win.

It isn't easy. To look inside and face yourself is something very few people, outside of those who elect to enter therapy, attempt to do. That's because it is far more comfortable to look at what we eat, focus on our genes, or search for medical excuses for obesity, than to deal with things that, in essence, comprise who we know ourselves to be.

For a long time I have known that the only way to permanently eliminate overeating is to eschew the popular myths offered us and instead harness the power of science. You now know that too, and if you are like me, you are going to want to talk about it.

Please E-mail or write to me, care of my publisher, Birch Lane Press, with your stories, comments, and questions. I will be delighted to hear from you and will be prompt to respond:

Dr. Cynthia G. Last
The 5 Reasons Why We Overeat
c/o Birch Lane Press
120 Enterprise Avenue
Secaucus, N.J. 07094

E-mail: CGLast@aol.com

I look forward to your stories.